Keith Mich

Practically

Macrobiotic

Cookbook

In this very special cookbook, Keith Michell, the internationally acclaimed award-winning actor, artist and author, draws aside the curtain of mystery that tends to obscure macrobiotics, and in his inimitably entertaining style shows that being practically macrobiotic doesn't mean a life of strict diets. Instead it is a way to enjoy to the full and gain health benefits from the vast variety of foodstuffs that nature supplies.

This book is excellent and informatively written . . . highly recommended.

Women and Home

An excellent introduction to a healthy lifestyle . . . delightful illustrations.

Journal of the Institute of Health Education

Rice

Keith Michell's Practically Macrobiotic Cookbook

Written and Illustrated by
Keith Michell

Healing Arts Press
Rochester, Vermont

Rice

Healing Arts Press
One Park Street
Rochester, Vermont 05767
www.InnerTraditions.com

Healing Arts Press is a division of Inner Traditions International

Note to the reader: This book is intended as an informational guide. The remedies, approaches, and techniques described herein are meant to supplement, and not to be a substitute for, professional medical care or treatment. They should not be used to treat a serious ailment without prior consultation with a qualified health care professional.

Library of Congress Cataloging-in-Publication Data

Michell, Keith.
     Keith Michell's practically macrobiotic cookbook / Keith Michell. — [Rev., expanded, and newly illustrated ed.]
     p.   cm.
Rev. ed. of: Practically macrobiotic / Keith Michell. 1987.
     Includes bibliographical references and index.
     ISBN 0-89281-848-4 (alk. paper)
     1. Macrobiotic diet Recipes. I. Michell, Keith. Practically macrobiotic cookbook.
RM235.M53   2000
641.5'63—dc21   99-40745
                                               CIP

Printed and bound in Hong Kong

10 9 8 7 6 5 4 3 2 1

Text design and layout by Priscilla Baker
This book was typeset in Hiroshige, with Calligraph as a display face.

Contents

Barley

It's a very odd thing—as odd as can be

That whatever Miss T eats turns into Miss T.

Walter de la Mare

Foreword

Following World War II, during the years 1945 to 1960, chemicalization, refinement, large-scale commercialization, and various types of artificialization of the food of the modern world became a standard. Trends leading to this state of affairs began in the early part of the twentieth century, together with the increased consumption of animal products, including red meat, poultry, and dairy food. At the same time, the use of refined sugar, as well as tropical and semitropical fruits and their juices, increased. While consumption of meat and sugar rose, use of whole cereal grains, beans and legumes, fresh vegetables, and locally grown fruits decreased.

With these dietary trends came changes in the health patterns of our societies. Degenerative diseases such as cardiovascular disorders, cancer, arthritis, allergies, diabetes, hypoglycemia, and many others, including psychological disorders such as schizophrenia, paranoia, depression, anxiety, and other emotional afflictions, have escalated as a result of these transitions into the modern world. Individual and family life has become more and more unstable; we are now witnessing massive decomposition of the family as a unit, increased crime and antisocial behavior, and a lack of cohesion in communities. These factors increase every year.

All of this indicates that modern society—in dietary habits, lifestyle, way of thinking, and other factors—is inadequate to sustain human health and maintain human spirituality on this planet.

For the past thirty years, the natural food movement, organic food movement, and holistic health advocates, especially those practicing the macrobiotic way of life, have been pioneering positive changes in diet, lifestyle, and way of thinking.

Modern macrobiotics, which draws upon the wisdom of ancient Greek, Judaic, and Oriental cultures and dietary practices, offers a positive solution for preventing various physical, psychological, and degenerative disorders, and offers possible recovery from them as well. Hundreds of thousands of people around the world who have begun the macrobiotic way of life have restored not only their physical health, but their psychological and spiritual health as well.

I take great pleasure in introducing *Keith Michell's Practically Macrobiotic*. The author, a well-known actor who has contributed greatly to humanity through his artistic expression, has compiled in this book many recipes for delicious and healthy macrobiotic and natural food dishes. Many of them are particularly helpful for those just beginning the macrobiotic approach, or for sharing with those friends who are unfamiliar with natural food cuisine. While some recipes contain foods not usually used in daily macrobiotic practice, especially during times of recovering one's health, they are helpful for those who are in transition to macrobiotics.

We wish to extend our sincere thanks to both the publisher and the author with our hope that this book may be read and used by many people who wish to maintain their health, prevent degenerative disorders, and recover their well-being.

Michio Kushi
Brookline, Mass., USA

Oats

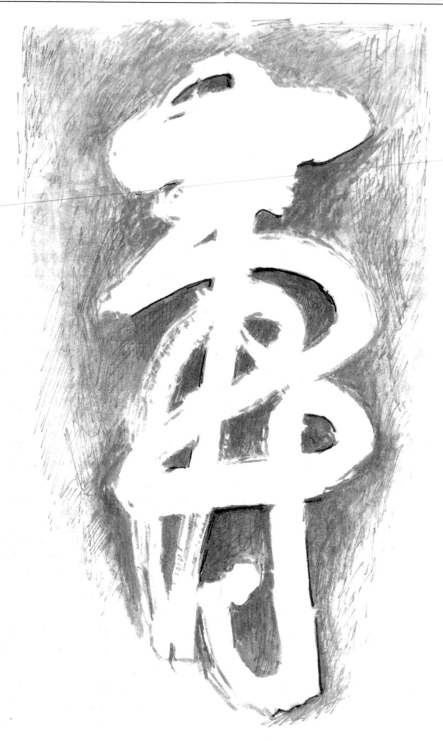

COPY OF THE CHARACTER *Shou (Long Life)*
IN *grass script* SIGNED BY THE 85 YEAR OLD
Yeh Chih. RUBBING DATED 1ST DAY OF THE 1ST MOON
1863

Introduction

Keith Michell has always put to best use an instinct for balance in his careers as artist and actor. No surprises, therefore, that he and macrobiotics should have embraced each other so closely. For macrobiotics is the way—or play—of harmony: the universal dynamics of change performed with graceful balance in our ever evolving lives.

This is a book of fine arts created by a fine artist of canvas and cuisine—to say nothing of his acting talents! One of the best things about helping Keith was being inspired by his wonderful illustrations, completed enthusiastically by him so early in the project. I sometimes felt we should be weaving a text around the pictures rather than merely illustrating the words. The worst thing has been having to keep the recipes secret for so long! When he first showed them to me, a year before publication, I casually remarked how well they would supplement the cooking courses I was running at the time. The look he gave me would have been familiar to several of Henry VIII's wives! It was a wise rebuke; exposure to the public then would surely have made the recipes the subject of untimely culinary espionage!

While it is true that the world needs new cooks more than another cookbook, there are still an astonishingly small number of recipe collections in which health aspects are not compromised by the regular palate placaters of dairy food and sugar. Twenty years ago, nutritional recommendations and macrobiotic dietary advice seemed poles apart; today they accommodate each other comfortably. Unsponsored voices in nutrition and medicine are calling for healthier diets based on whole grains, vegetables, seeds, nuts, and fruit, and with a strong emphasis on reducing meat, dairy foods, and sugar to minimal levels. But still there remains massive ignorance about nutrition and diet, often (unforgivably) among the medical profession. This despite the dawning realization in the health sciences that malnutrition is now the most widespread background health disorder in our "developed" world.

It was with a sense of urgency more than novelty, therefore, that Keith decided to incorporate nutritional explanations and data into a book about macrobiotics. This has not been easy to do for several reasons. Science and macrobiotics view food from different perspectives. The quality of "energy" (ch'i or ki) that is attributed to food in macrobiotics is not detected by nutritional analysis. For example, it is quite possible for a long-frozen sample of cabbage to show up equally as well in laboratory analysis as the freshly picked version. We know instinctively that fresh is best for us. Nutrition doesn't. Food composition values are interesting and useful as long as they are not taken too literally. The data provided here will at least reveal how rich in nutrients and low in harmful aspects is the macrobiotic way of eating. A recent London University study shows that the macrobiotic diet is adequate in all nutrients and is full of those nutrients often lacking in the modern diet.

Millet

Macrobiotics has had quite a rough ride until recently. Misunderstandings and poor translations in the early days of its introduction to the West attracted a tiny but lunatic fringe of zealots who chose to interpret this gentle way of harmony as a kind of metabolic martial art—on one or two occasions even extinguishing themselves in the process. Secular medical judgment was, not surprisingly, fairly hysterical, which served only to compound the misunderstanding and delay progress toward a more "westernized" application of macrobiotic dietary principles. New research by Belgian doctors into the blood chemistry and tissue function of macrobiotic men and children has revealed a perfect picture of health. Other recent medical studies are similarly supportive.

As governments are at last being forced by public opinion to take real interest in preventive health care, official recommendations for healthy eating are showing some hopeful trends. We should not, however, be complacent enough to believe that politicians in power hold the health of the people dearer to their hearts than they do the pressing attentions of the food, drug, and agriculture industries. It is we, as individuals, groups, and communities, who must spread the message—at least until it is received and understood by a critical mass of society. For the food/health connection is an absolutely crucial issue at this stage of humanity's journey, much as were health and hygiene in relation to the killer epidemics of the nineteenth century.

The health of westerners has degenerated in this century to levels that would permit few of us to survive in the lifestyles of even our most recent ancestors. Modern medicine has little of use to offer beyond powerful painkillers and some effective emergency care. It continues to foster a mentality that seeks to blame illness on factors "beyond our control," rather than teaching us to accept responsibility for our disease and thus to learn something from it: but these latter days of the twentieth century are drawing us through the funnel of transformation into a brighter age. We have no alternative but to make this journey successfully, and we should be prepared to face a good deal of turbulence on the way. At this time our most valuable resource is sound health of body, mind, and spirit.

How can macrobiotics help us in our progression? To move into a healthier future we need to rid ourselves of a sick past, abolish old fears, and build with the vision of uncluttered consciousness.

Macrobiotics does help transform worn-down health into welcome new potentials. It plays a powerful role in dissolving and eliminating the consequences of inappropriate habits accumulated in tissues, organs, muscles, and joints through years of dietary and mental self-abuse. And it makes us feel good!—about ourselves, the world around us, and our relationship with it.

Finally, and most importantly, macrobiotic food is delicious! At the risk of evoking another goodbye look from Keith I must admit to having tested these recipes, albeit in intimate company and in a far-off land. They are wonderful—among the best I have ever found. As you explore and enjoy them, please remember to give thanks that food of such quality, variety, and goodness is available to be shared among us.

Richard Burton BSc
London, England

Introducing Macrobiotics

And What Is Your Favorite Food?

Macrobi-what-ics?

So You Expect to Live to a Hundred, Do You?

Who Started It All?

And What Is Your Favorite Food?

There is no doubt that the subject of food can be a delicate one. In interviews, when a question like "And what is your favorite food?" is innocently asked, and a word like *macrobiotics* is uttered, interviewers tend to look startled. They could have a crank on their hands—a possibly dangerous one—who might try to convert them!

Let me say at once that I do not pretend to be an authority on the subject of macrobiotics. I don't think of myself as a cook—neither does anyone else as far as I know—and I never try to convert anyone. I'm not a particularly rigid practicing macrobiotic, which is probably the best sort to be. There are more extensive books written on the philosophy of the subject and several fine cookbooks. I am indebted to the authors of both categories. I eat my own *practically* macrobiotic way because I enjoy it. Being asked to write this book (and now to revise it for a new edition) has been a good opportunity to find answers to many of the questions asked by interviewers, skeptics, and friends over the past twenty-five years and, I might add, a chance to answer quite a few I have needed to ask myself about macrobiotics.

Macrobi-what-ics?

The word (it is *macrobiotics*, by the way, not *microbiotics*) does conjure up the science laboratory rather than the humble kitchen, but it is not exactly a science because it is founded in philosophy. It is neither a cult nor a religion, but it can contribute to a good way of life. There are probably as many different interpretations of it as there are people who practice it.

Oats

Basically it is a practical way of selecting, preparing, cooking, and eating food—not necessarily with chopsticks—based on the ancient and beautiful concept of Tao.

Tao is "the pursuit of the *natural* way of heaven and Earth—the order of the universe; the Great Whole, containing all change."

The Chinese have a symbol or character called *shou*, which means longevity. This could be the origin of the word *macrobiotics*. The Greek translation of *shou* is *macro*, long (or great) and *biotic*, meaning life. (*Microbiotics*, on the other hand, means small or short life!)

So You Expect to Live to a Hundred, Do You?

Our body will survive on a physical level anywhere from forty to a hundred years however badly or well we treat it—but who wants a long life if it is a miserable or painful one? Personally I prefer the "Great Life" translation, in which it is not the quantity of life that is important but the quality of it. Whether it is *macro*, great, or generally unsatisfactory is up to us.

Have you ever considered how meticulous we are about the fuel we feed our automobiles? Our bodies, on the other hand, are such infinitely more sophisticated pieces of machinery that by comparison even a satellite would seem as simple as a covered wagon. Yet we go on stuffing them with any junk we can find in the supermarket without so much as a glance at the labels.

One consequence of this treatment is that the use of tranquilizers alone has reached "epidemic proportions" according to a National Association of Mental Health report. One person in seven of the United Kingdom adult population takes these drugs every year.

What we eat and drink affects us physically, mentally, and certainly spiritually. This is such a statement of the obvious and so simple that we tend to overlook it. Occasionally a hangover brutally brings the fact to our attention or sickness makes us recognize it. Both signal to us the fact that we are not eating naturally. Mind you, these days it is almost impossible to find food, water, salt, or even air in its natural unadulterated state! Realizing this danger is halfway to dealing with it.

I was forcibly made aware of the importance of food when, in Australia as a teenager, just learning to stand on my own two feet, I landed in a hospital bed with a serious attack of tonsillitis—and a throat so inflamed and swollen that I couldn't swallow. The effects of the illness were soon cured by injections of the latest drug—penicillin—and the doctor threatened to remove the offending tonsils as soon as the patient's condition improved. Fortunately, a far-seeing friend advised a visit to a naturopath instead. This man explained that the tonsils are one of nature's many ingenious warning devices used by the body to indicate an excess of toxins in the system. He advised cutting down on chocolates, cakes, sugary sweets, and food fried in lard. It made sense.

Two decades or so later—1970—and the scene is New York, that city where a "healthy" diet can consist of synthetic food and vitamin pills. I was healthy enough—greedy but healthy and showing some signs of being overweight—but I seemed to have a continual hangover from which I never quite recovered. The food served in most restaurants was certainly boring. The menus were monotonous, overelaborate, overcooked, and overpriced.

Then I was given a book as a joke, *You Are All Sanpaku* by William Dufty, about a man named George Ohsawa and his macrobiotics. It was a bestseller.

I was back in England trying out a new play before I got around to reading the book. Dufty, the author, had had every complaint you could think of, from headaches to hemorrhoids, and cured them all by this practical way of eating devised by Ohsawa. The book made startling, thundering sense to me. "You are what you eat," it said. "Physical and mental disorder comes from a disordered, unnatural way of eating."

The play settled down for a London run, and I settled down to eating "macrobiotically." This meant eating mainly brown rice and mixed vegetables with some fish and prawns, "real" soy sauce and sesame salt, no sugar or sugar products, and drinking less liquid. After three days I started losing weight—twenty pounds in ten days—and I could see muscles and things I'd forgotten I had! Best of all was a relaxation and mental clarity—a "high" you might say. Only I was kicking "drugs," namely sugar and chemicals, which gave me a strange new awareness and lack of anxiety—call it happiness—I hadn't experienced in years.

By the time we took the play to Los Angeles I was getting thin. My leading lady, Diana Rigg, remarked in her inimitable way that the audience wouldn't see me at all in our nude scene if I didn't do something about it! Actually I was the same weight I had been in my twenties.

I looked up the address of the Ohsawa Foundation and went along to ask a few questions. A woman there gave an hour of her time and some valuable advice. *Eat what you feel like but always remember the balance of yin and yang.* She said, "Cooking techniques from other countries, especially the Orient, can seem strange. Westerners are not used to the cooking methods, and eating nothing but rice and sea vegetables, however well cooked, seems a sacrifice which perhaps the body is not prepared to accept. It can, in fact, be dangerous to suddenly go on a diet of grains. If you feel like eating a steak do so—with green vegetables and a glass of wine to balance it! Just be aware of the balance. Above all, don't become a fanatic about it."

At the time Johnny (Tarzan) Weissmuller had a health shop named after him on Hollywood Boulevard, and there I found three of Ohsawa's original volumes. In his *Macrobiotic Guide Book* Ohsawa says the same thing: "Some people think that macrobiotics is no more than the eating of sesame seeds mixed with sea salt, carrots, and brown rice. Others that it is summed up by 'Don't eat cake and sugar.' How far from the truth! . . . I enjoy any cuisine—Western, Chinese, Japanese, Indian. I like fruit, candy, chocolate and whisky very much. If I choose to use these things now I am able to avoid harm because I can balance the yin and yang. We must choose what is good for us—the art of making such a choice is macrobiotics."

I have stayed with this way of eating—or my interpretation of it—for twenty-five years or more now, mainly for practical reasons. It is easy to prepare, tastes good, and has stood me in good stead. An actor's life can be as vigorous and as stressful as an athlete's—physical and emotional demands and mental disciplines can be a heavier strain than people realize. More important, I love the grub and the way it makes me feel!

I really prefer grains to meat as a principal food. *Whole* grains, that is. There's such a choice! Millet is a good food, as are oats, barley, rye, wheat, buckwheat, corn, and, of course, the good old standby, rice. I don't mean the cotton wool flakes of what is called "refined" rice but rich, chewy, short-grained brown rice. Seasonal vegetables in both England and the United States are superb, and seaweeds or sea vegetables such as laver, dulse, carrageen, and kelp eaten in parts of Europe are a rich source of minerals not as yet generally appreciated. There are a thousand new tastes to discover. Ohsawa says the food tastes of nature, and he's right! It is very exciting and never bland—unless it's badly cooked.

And in this day and age of neuroses and violence, macrobiotics helps bring some balance to life itself—the yin and yang balance of nature.

In this book I have tried to give you an idea of the sort of food there is to enjoy, new ingredients and recipes not only from the East but from other parts of the world. Most traditional dishes were originally macrobiotic when they were made from unrefined, whole ingredients and were balanced by man's and woman's intuition. Over the centuries, grains have long been the principal food of most civilizations, with vegetables, legumes or beans and, from time to time, some animal products, fish or meat, as supplements.

For those who are nervous about their vitamins, minerals, protein, and so forth, there are lists of nutrient content of *whole* foods included. Nutritionists approach the subject of diet analytically and scientifically but are, you will find, continually confirming the common sense of macrobiotics.

Assembling the material for this book has been one of life's adventures I would not have missed! I am grateful to John Hardaker of Thorsons Publishing Group for suggesting I write it and for his encouragement. I said yes to the idea without quite realizing what would be involved, and it wasn't long before a long overdue visit was paid to the Community Health Foundation at the East West Centre, Old Street, London. There they quickly summed me up as an "old-fashioned macrobiotic!" I'd like to thank those members of the foundation—Anna McKenzie, Montse and Peter Bradford, Lynne Stackhouse, and Alastaire G. Drane for bringing my wife, Jenny, and me up-to-date on the latest developments in the yin-yang kitchen. There are many new products on the market that make the cooking even more exciting, and many refinements of preparation I have tried to include in the following chapters. Jenny brings her own continental flair to cooking and, I am glad to say, patiently keeps me off the *too* straight and narrow culinary path by insisting on varying the menus.

Working in the theater meant traveling to the United States and Australia last year—equipped with pots, pans, and *suribachi*. This is why the illustrations are done with felt pens. They are easy to pack and light to carry!

While rehearsing in New York we discovered a popular macrobiotic restaurant run by a young Englishman, Richard Markstein, who has great enthusiasm for and belief in the potential of macrobiotics. In San Francisco we found a young Argentinian, Louis Gutman, whose love for cooking and understanding of macrobiotics was remarkable. Both Richard and Louis generously contributed some of their own special recipes to this collection and encountering their freshness of spirit, which so many young macrobiotics seem to have, was a great pleasure. In Australia Brian and Anne Perkins and Suzan and Stefan Melkonian provided some fine meals and recipes with an Antipodean flavor.

I am particularly indebted to Richard Burton, BSc, then nutritionist with the London Community Health Foundation; apart from his encouragement, Richard has painstakingly revised the text and has written a foreword to it. I would like to mention Angela Piscina, who has bravely applied her considerable skills experimenting with new dishes and ingredients; Roger Watson, Ph.D. who has shared culinary secrets and offered valuable advice; and Bernie Echevarri who expertly deciphered and typed innumerable handwritten drafts with hardly a demur. There are others—they will know who they are—who have provided help, recipes, and encouragement. I thank them for their contribution to this book, which will, I hope, serve as an introduction to the subject of macrobiotics. Finally, I thank Ehud Sperling and those at Inner Traditions for their faith in this book and for publishing a new edition of it.

Who Started It All?

The first to use the word *macrobiotics* seems to have been a physician, Christopher Wilhelm Hufeland, who worked in Berlin and wrote a book called *Macrobiotik—The Art of Prolonging Human Life*. This was 150 years before George Ohsawa was to apply it in connection with food, cooking, and Tao. Ohsawa also apparently introduced and first practiced acupuncture in Europe. He also brought the spirit of the Tao and of judo and kadu (flower arrangement) to the West.

To read his books is to encounter a somewhat stern, righteous, Eastern prophet proclaiming to the Western wilderness, in sometimes quaint English, his fervent faith in health or hell on Earth. This, I suppose, is pretty much what he was.

Early this century he was a young Oriental student, and the East was becoming westernized. At that time natural whole food certainly hadn't the ring of sound common sense it has today, nor was the situation of refined, convenience food as serious as it has more recently become. George Bernard Shaw advocated vegetarianism and was considered a crank, but then so had Buddha, Pythagoras, Plato, Plutarch, Ovid, Seneca, Milton, Pope, Shelley, Voltaire, Rousseau, Tolstoy, Newton, and Gandhi! Obviously a thinking man's diet! Macrobiotics is, to my mind, a logical and natural progression from vegetarianism.

Ohsawa came from a westernized Japanese family and found his healthy way of eating through sickness. In fact he nearly died when he was only sixteen. His young mother, sisters, and brothers were victims of tuberculosis, and he too was condemned as incurable by his Western doctors. As a "poor orphan" he said he could no longer afford their treatment anyway. This was fortunate for him because he turned to a Japanese doctor in Tokyo, Sagan Ishizuka.

In those days nutrition was mainly concerned with the three organic ingredients—protein, fat, and carbohydrate—but in Ishizuka's opinion the body's functions, organs, and nervous system were controlled by the *inorganic minerals,* in particular, potassium and sodium, and he divided foods into those two categories. Foods, he claimed, were the highest medicines, and all physical characteristics such as skin texture, overweight/underweight, good memory or bad, strength or weakness depended on environment *and* the intake of potassium and sodium. He wrote a book called *Chemical Diet for Longevity* and became very famous. A letter addressed to "Dr. Antidoctor, Tokyo" was delivered directly to him.

He cured Ohsawa, who studied his theory, related it to Oriental philosophy, and realized that a concept explaining it has existed in the Orient for two thousand years. He lived to launch his macrobiotics, and for over fifty years advocated his reinterpretation of the "unique principle" of Tao as a basis for healthier and more peaceful living. Macrobiotics, he claimed, was a simple, practical discipline of life that anyone could practice with great pleasure to help restore health and harmony of soul, mind, and body. "The theory is so simple," he wrote, "a child can learn it. There is only one principle to understand—*yin and yang—a universal compass, the heart of a world concept which can be applied throughout our daily life on every level.*"

During World War II Ohsawa was imprisoned in Japan for his antiwar activities. In 1946 he helped form the World Government Association in Hiyoshi under the splendid title of Center Ignoramus, where the principle of yin and yang was taught. In 1952 he and his wife, Lima, started traveling. They stayed in India, lived with Dr. Schweitzer in Africa, then moved to France and Belgium teaching macrobiotics. In 1961 they went to the United States and established the Ohsawa Foundation in

California, where his books were published. The clinic he ran was called Sanrant: *Sanatorium* + res-tau*rant*. There was no operating theater, no drug department: its center was the kitchen. "In macrobi-otics our pharmacy is the kitchen," he wrote. "Our method is based on the potency of daily food."

His life was spent interpreting Oriental philosophy; and more than anything he wished to bring West and East together. This, as he saw it, was the world's chief hope of peace and freedom—two mighty words—which only faith in man's oneness with nature could achieve. Having taught his meth-ods for fifty years, he admitted that although he was convinced of its great value, there was still a chance that he might be wrong. "Why otherwise," he asked, "in all these years have I been able to find so few Western doctors or philosophers who can understand the writing and philosophy that were taken for granted in the East centuries ago?"

Time seems to be answering his question. Nearly thirty years after his death the spirit of macrobi-otics—the oneness of humanity, nature, and the universe, seems to be surviving! Yin and yang are being integrated into Western thinking. After some initial vehement resistance, Oriental philosophy is influencing Occidental medical treatments, nutrition, and what we eat perhaps more than Ohsawa ever imagined it would and more than we ourselves realize. In recent years the great increase in the number of shops supplying health products throughout England, the United States and parts of Eu-rope and Australia is a response to public dissatisfaction and demand. Most such shops, even super-markets, successfully stock macrobiotic supplies. Natural eating is definitely coming back!

Everything changes and, as I discovered in those cooking classes, the concepts of macrobiotics are continually being revised to suit other new decades. Our scientists' ventures into space have accustomed us to universal awareness and, according to Michio Kushi, Ohsawa's successor, macrobi-otics is a way of life according to the largest possible view. "One day," he says, "future generations will look back at the cult of our modern civilization's artificial food as a fad . . . under many names and forms macrobiotics will continue as long as human life continues to exist."

A Postscript to the Revised Edition

Over the fifteen years since this book was first published, it has been interesting to watch the media, dieticians, and medical advisors in general, gradually apply the principles of Ohsawa. In the 1960s the use of the word *organic* indicated a certain eccentricity. When writing this book in the 1980s I sug-gested organic food with reservation—it was scarce, expensive, and suspect. Now, however, organic products are demanded by consumers and are being stocked even by most supermarkets—certainly by those in the UK and Europe.

Recently in England there have been demonstrations and outcries condemning the genetic engi-neering of food. These have been triggered by a nightmare scenario in which giant multinational cor-porations have been given free rein to add or subtract genetic materials that alter the organisms in our food chain. Such genetic engineering is an unpredictable, inaccurate, and dangerous science. Hap-hazard experiments have been carried out without proper safety testing or regard for environmental protection, even without our knowledge. The resulting products have been, without warning and unla-beled, quietly slipped onto our supermarket shelves.

It is only by insisting on buying organic food that we consumers can continue to apply economic pressure and send a strong message to the biotech companies that genetic products are not wanted in our kitchens. Read your labels and insist that your food is grown naturally.

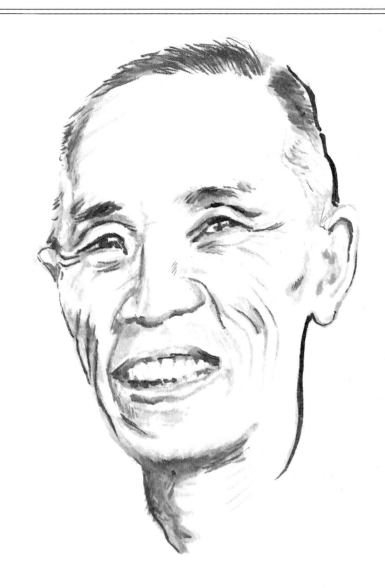

Accept everything with great pleasure and thanks. ACCEPT MISFORTUNE LIKE HAPPINESS, DISEASE LIKE HEALTH, POVERTY LIKE PROSPERITY. and if you don't like it or cannot stand it, refer to your UNIVERSAL COMPASS the UNIQUE PRINCIPLE. There you will find the best direction. Everything that happens to you is what you lack. all that is ANTAGONISTIC, unbearable is COMPLIMENTARY THE MAN WHO EMBRACES HIS ANTAGONIST IS THE HAPPIEST MAN — George Ohsawa.

Yin and Yang

Yin and Yang are the two arms of the Infinite, the Absolute Oneness—God.

Yin and Yang are continuous, forever in motion and changing.

Yin attracts yang: yang attracts yin.

Yin repels yin: yang repels yang.

Yin-yang components are constantly changing.

Nothing is completely yin or completely yang.

Either yin exceeds yang or yang exceeds yin.

Nothing is neutral.

Yin and Yang together produce all energy.

All opposites are complementary.

There can be no front without a back,

no beauty without ugliness.

What Is This Yin and Yang??

The question requires an answer. Now *that* is yin and yang!

The diagram on page 12 shows yin and yang as complementary opposites that together make a whole. Understanding this, the Unique Principle, is what Tao is all about. "Wholeness," said George Ohsawa, "is the highest wisdom . . . everything can be understood the better through an awareness of this harmony of opposites."

We in the West tend to think of natural opposition as absolute and separate. Good *versus* bad, rich *versus* poor, left wing *versus* right wing. But yin and yang coexist as two sides of oneness, of the universe—of God or what you will.

The earliest idea of complementary opposites was probably that of the Earth Mother—the Tellus Mater—who provided life by her fertility, and of the Sky Father, who controlled the sun and elements necessary for growth and fertilization. In Greek mythology there were Chaos and Earth. According to Indian mythology Shiva is the destroyer—the male power—and Vishnu the preserver, the female power. In the beautiful Chinese Book of Changes, the *I Ching*, Ch'ien represents the sky power, Father and Heaven, while K'un is the yielding Mother and Earth. To the ancient Chinese the calm, receptive, peaceful, and earthly powers were yin. Strength, aggression, violence, and clamor were heavenly powers and yang!

Yin and yang. The Mother and Father who bring about all changes. These forces are still discussed quite seriously today in Somerset, where the Glastonbury Tor is set in the Valley of Avalon. It is a mysterious, spiraling mound, the center of a vast "round table" with its Glastonbury Giants spread for miles around—zodiac symbols so large that they are visible only from the air. Sun-God-Sagittarius (King Arthur) and Earth-Mother-Virgo (Guinevere) are outlined by natural contours, roads, and waterways. Were they conjured up by nature across the landscape or by the power of Celtic mythology and humanity's fertile imagination?

Yin and yang are equally important, let me hasten to add! Each has its natural place. They can only survive in relationship; they mutually attract, depend on, and influence one another. Neither is totally yin nor completely yang. They achieve oneness in the natural order of things. The yin-yang of female and male, the passive-receptive and active-creative energies are only one tiny balance on the mighty scale. The number of yin-yang opposites is infinite.

You will find yin and yang everywhere, at all times. Breathing out follows breathing in, expansion eases contraction, separates gather together, silence quiets sound, stillness stays activity, outward embraces inward, negative discharges positive, weakness shall overcome strength, high rests upon low, water quenches fire, shadow is cast by light, striving up touches bearing down, day is changed by night, space is measured by time. They oppose and complement each other and will eventually mutually transform each other. Summer changes to winter, youth to age, matter to energy. Every beginning has an end. Yin and yang. Even the colors of the spectrum are a facet of it. The cooler colors of yin—purples, blues, and greens—contrast their complements, the warmer reds, oranges, and yellows which are yang. Together they make light.

Foods are also carriers of these two powerful forces, and when we eat food we produce cells, muscles, nerves, hormones, enzymes, genes, organs, and thoughts that are antagonistic and complementary. Both yin foods and yang foods are needed by our bodies. Being aware of this provides a quite remarkable compass when cooking! Yin and yang balance seems to help maintain a balance in one's attitudes, too.

Try it and see. Your body—and your mind—will be grateful.

So Which Foods Are Yin and Which Are Yang?

There are a number of factors that influence the yin-yang of food. Generally speaking, as you see in the chart on page 13, fruits and vegetables are more yin, grains and legumes more balanced (slightly yin), animal products more yang. You can eat more or less what you wish, but avoid extremes of yin or yang whenever possible.

The old maxim "You are what you eat" is so astonishingly simple that the usual reaction is to joke about it. But take a good, hard look at people who are compulsive pork or beef eaters! Meat is an elaborate, expensive, and painful (not only for the animal!) way to obtain protein that is available directly from grains and beans. I am convinced that most of the senseless violence in the world is caused by the growing fad of prosperous societies who insist on meals predominantly comprising animal flesh every day.

In time you will come to judge food quality for yourself. Being aware of yin-yang properties can help you to recognize their presence in food, and you will enjoy the yin-yang experience.

CENTRIFUGAL

CONTRACTING

DOWNWARDS

HIGHER

LIGHTER WEIGHT

EXPANDING

CENTRIPETAL

MALE

MORE AGGRESSIVE

ACTIVE PHYSICAL

HARDER

WARMER

OUTWARD

UPWARDS

INWARD

COLDER

SOFTER

MORE RECEPTIVE

PASSIVE MENTAL

FEMALE

Yang

△

HEAVIER WEIGHT

LOWER

faster
fire
drier
brighter
proton
longer wave
positive charge
time

slower
water
wetter
darker
electron
shorter wave
negative charge
space

Yin

▽

RED   ORANGE   YELLOW

GREEN   BLUE   INDIGO   VIOLET

SALTY · BITTER

SLOWER COOKING

LESS SMELL

MORE DRY

HARDER

SMALLER

SLOWER GROWTH

DRIER SOIL

GROWN IN COOLER CLIMATE

grown on ground

VERTICAL GROWTH DOWNWARDS

CEREALS

ANIMAL

MORE COOKED

RAW VEGETABLE SALADS

VERTICAL GROWTH UPWARDS

grown on tree

GROWN IN HOTTER CLIMATE

DAMPER SOIL

FASTER GROWTH

LARGER

SOFTER

MORE JUICE

STRONGER SMELL

FASTER COOKING

SPICY · SOUR · SWEET

more Yang

more Sodium & other yang elements
lower fat content
faster moving (animal)
warm body temperature

more Yin

more potassium & yin elements
higher fat content
stationary (vegetable)
cooler temperature

Generally speaking, whatever contains water is more yin. However, there are other indications of yin and yang. Colors can help identification: violet, indigo, blue, green, or white show yin, while yellow, orange, red, and brown or black generally show more yang. (There are exceptions—tomatoes are red and extremely yin!) The taste can range from yin-spicy, sour, and sweet to yang-salty and bitter. Fat and protein content makes for yin, carbohydrate and mineral content for yang.

Fruits and vegetables, being more yin, grow upward and expansively. Their effect on body temperature is cooling: Those that have violet, blue, green, or white colors are more yin, and those with yellow, orange, brown, or red colors are usually more yang. Those grown in hot, tropical regions are more yin than are those grown in the colder climates. They tend to have a stronger odor and taste, to be juicier and softer, to grow faster and cook more quickly, which are properties of yin.

Vegetables grown in spring and summer are more yin than those grown in autumn and winter. If they grow vertically and expansively above the earth they are more yin than those growing under the earth and downward. Carrots, for example, are orange in color, are harder, drier, more compact, and more yang than most vegetables, but are more yin than grains.

Grains are very small and compact, ripen slowly, are dry, hard and brown, gold or yellow in color, with little odor or taste. They are more yang than are most other vegetables but are more yin than meat.

Animal products are much more yang. They form separate, compact units with a more compact inward formation of organs and cells. They have warm body temperatures, and they move about, some faster (the more yang ones) than others. Their color is generally that of hemoglobin (yang) red.

White, cold-blooded fish, shellfish, and so on are less yang than are warm-blooded meat and fowl. Freshwater fish are less yang than saltwater fish.

Vegetables being more yin tend to produce a more overall relaxation in the body's functions. Animal products, on the other hand, being more yang, make for tenseness. Yin foods and yang foods are complementary, and they mutually attract. If you eat salty (yang) food, you will tend to crave sweets (yin).

Ideally, food should be mainly grain and vegetable quality, selected from the middle of the yin-yang scale.

Yin and yang correspond to the seasons. In spring and summer in hot, tropical climates we tend to eat more yin foods. We prefer salads, lightly cooked vegetables, and some fruit as dessert. Because hot weather is yang, we need the yin food as a balance, and nature supplies it. In cooler seasons like autumn and winter in cold climates, we crave more yang foods—grains such as millet, buckwheat, short-grained rice, root vegetables, slightly more salt, and even some animal products. These help warm us and keep out the cold.

Always try to buy vegetables in season or grown in your own geographical area if possible. They are cheaper then anyway, because they are more plentiful. In this day and age of export and import, choose your vegetables from a climate similar to your own or from the same latitude. Treat those exotic delicacies from the tropics with some restraint. Such foods are yin and will cool you down, which you don't need in the middle of a freezing winter. They make you feel cold and generally prevent your body from adapting to your natural weather conditions.

Cooking affects yin and yang. Cooking can transform a meal. Grains, beans, vegetables, seaweeds, and nuts—some more yin than others—may need to be made more yang, especially in winter or in a cold climate. Fire, pressure, salt, and time are the chief yang factors. Baking, roasting, grilling, pressure cooking, sautéing, and the use of sea salt, tamari, miso, and pickles all help to yangize and energize food. Meat, shellfish, and poultry need less yang treatment. Boiling, steaming, and the use of fresh salads, some spices, fruit, and desserts help yinize a meal. Raw fish is less extreme yang than is cooked (see INGREDIENTS—Sashimi). Cooking is the art of adjusting these factors and adapting food to the season, time, and place and the needs of the individual. When you know your yin from your yang you will enjoy balancing a meal, and you and yours will feel a great deal better for it.

Do Yin and Yang Mean Acid and Alkaline?

This question is often asked, and the answer is yes—and no!

When Ohsawa studied Ishizuka's theory that sodium and potassium were the most important inorganic minerals in the body, and related it to the Unique Principle and Tao, he realized that he needed to categorize acid and alkaline in relation to yin and yang. In what was probably his first book, *Lecture Series in Shokuyo*, published in 1928, he called acid yang and alkaline yin. By the sixties, however, when he first lectured in New York, acid had become yin and alkaline yang. Yin or potassium-containing foods were acidic, he claimed, and yang or sodium-containing foods were alkaline. He set the desirable ratio of yin (potassium) and yang (sodium) at something between 3:1 and 7:1.

But potassium and sodium are two metallic elements with such very similar characteristics that it is often difficult to tell them apart—and both are alkaline! Once in the body, however, as electrically charged ions, they are completely complementary *and* antagonistic to one another. Their yin-yang relationship is essential to the body's proper functioning.

Nutritionists, however, talk about two types of food. First, acid or alkaline foods—how acidic or alkaline the *food* is. Second, acid- and alkaline-*forming* foods—the condition the foods cause in the body after they are eaten. Biochemically, the chief alkaline-producing elements are calcium, potassium, sodium, and magnesium. These balance the main acid-forming elements of phosphorus, sulfur, and chlorine. The alkaline-producing elements keep the blood and intercellular fluids alkaline, in spite of the body's continuous metabolic production of large amounts of acid.

High protein foods, and especially animal products, contain abundant quantities of sulfur and phosphorus, which in the body are acid forming.

Grains also contain some sulfur and phosphorus, and most of them are considered acid forming.

Most fruits and vegetables contain potassium, sodium, calcium, and magnesium. They may have a sharp "acidic" taste—but they neutralize body acid!

Ohsawa never classified the difference between acid-forming and alkaline-forming foods, but Herman Aihara sums it up in his book on the subject: "The characteristics of acid and alkali are very similar to the Oriental concept of Yin and Yang—which is a whole concept of life. Yin and Yang are always changing in our life just as acid and alkali work in us."

Ohsawa classified the yin-yang of elements by using spectroscopy. All elements radiate specific wavelengths: longwave radiation is yang, and shortwave is yin. According to Ohsawa, sodium has a longwave radiation and is therefore yang, while potassium produces shortwave (yin) radiation. The spectroscopic colors are interesting—sodium is orange (yang) and potassium violet (yin):

Yin ▽

Fruits

TROPICAL
LEMONS
PEACHES
PEARS
ORANGES, LIMES
WATER MELON
APPLES, CHERRIES
STRAWBERRIES

Beverages

SUGARED DRINKS
FRUIT JUICES
COFFEE
DYED TEAS
MINERAL WATERS
SODA WATER
WELL WATER
HERBAL TEAS
KOKKOH
DANDELION ROOT
BANCHA TEA
BURDOCK ROOT
MU TEA
GINSENG ROOT

Alcoholic Beverages

VODKA
WINE
CHAMPAGNE
WHISKY
SAKE
BEER

Vegetables

POTATOES
EGGPLANT TOMATOES
SHIITAKE PEPPERS
CUCUMBER
SWEET PEPPERS
SPINACH
ASPARAGUS
ARTICHOKE
BAMBOO SHOOTS
MUSHROOMS
RED CABBAGE, BEET
BRUSSELS SPROUTS
CAULIFLOWER
BROCCOLI, CABBAGE
DANDELION LEAF
LETTUCE, ENDIVE, KALE
ONION, GARLIC
PARSNIP, TURNIP.
DAIKON RADISH
LEEKS
PUMPKIN SQUASH
MARROW COURGETTE
WATERCRESS
BURDOCK
DANDELION ROOT
CARROT
JENINJO

Dairy Foods

ICE CREAM
YOGHURT
MILK

GOAT'S MILK

SOFT CHEESES
HARD CHEESES

Sea Vegetables

NORI
HIZIKI
WAKAME
KOMBU

Nuts & Seeds

CASHEWS
PEANUTS
ALMONDS
CHESTNUTS

SQUASH SEEDS
PUMPKIN SEEDS
SUNFLOWER SEEDS
SESAME SEEDS

Beans

SOYA BEANS
GREEN PEAS
WHITE
PINTO
KIDNEY
LENTILS
BLACK
CHICK PEAS
AZUKI

Grains

CORN
OATS
BARLEY
RYE
WHEAT
RICE
MILLET
BUCKWHEAT

Animal Food

SHELL FISH
WHITE MEAT FISH
FOWL
MEAT
RED MEAT FISH
EGGS

Condiments

GOMASIO
TEKKA

TAMARI
MISO

SALT

Yang ▲

This chart, showing the yin-yang relation between the various food categories, is adapted from Ohsawa's original table.

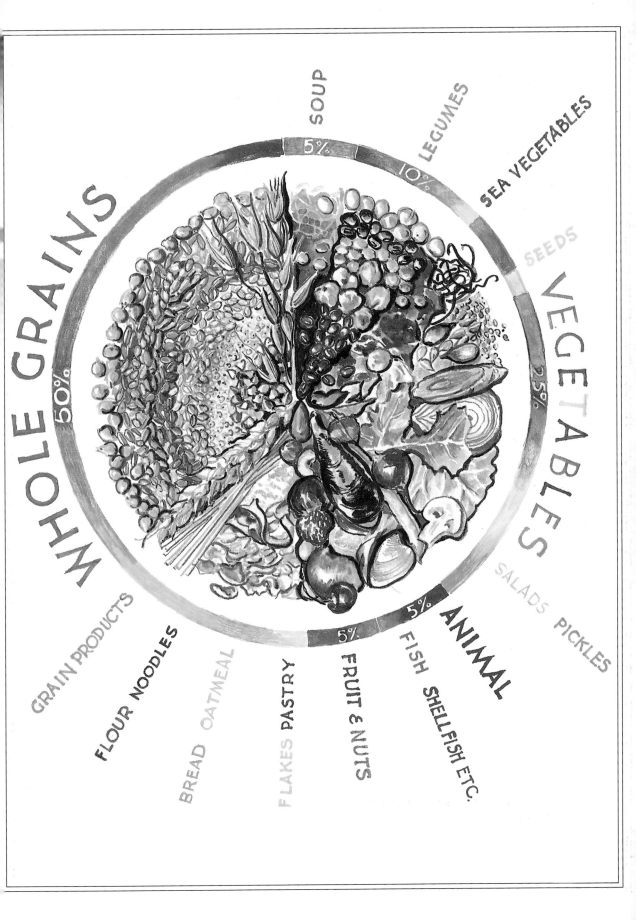

WHOLE GRAINS 50%

GRAIN PRODUCTS FLOUR NOODLES BREAD OATMEAL FLAKES PASTRY FRUIT & NUTS

SOUP 5%

LEGUMES 10%

SEA VEGETABLES

SEEDS

VEGETABLES 25%

SALADS PICKLES

ANIMAL 5%

FISH SHELLFISH ETC.

5%

Yin and Yang

RED	ORANGE	YELLOW	GREEN	BLUE	VIOLET
6500Å					4289Å
Hydrogen					
Carbon	Sodium				
		Magnesium		Oxygen	Nitrogen
		Chlorine		Phosphorus	
				Sulfur	
				Calcium	Potassium
					Manganese
				Iron	
			Copper		

YANG ACTIVITY————————————————————————————YIN ACTIVITY

Ishizuka and Ohsawa set the ideal ratio of potassium to sodium in human food at 5:1. It is interesting to note that in a list of food compositions published by Ohsawa in 1938 rice was considered to have the perfect balance of yin and yang; the potassium-sodium ratio was K23:Na4.6, that is, 5:1. In 1970 this ratio, according to "Food Values of Portions Commonly Used," Bowes and Church, had changed to K112:Na9, that is, 12:1. Two other sources, including the United States Department of Agriculture, give the potassium-sodium ratio of rice as K214:Na9, which is nearly 24:1! Herman Aihara conjectures that this increase in potassium may be because foods are now much more yin as a result of the fertilizers and chemicals used to grow them.

Putting a Meal Together

Soup, approximately 5 percent

Grains, 50 percent or more

Legumes (and Seeds), more or less 10 percent

Vegetables (and Sea Vegetables), about 25 percent

Animal Products, 5 percent or no more than 10 percent

Seasoning

Desserts, Fruits, and Nuts, a moderate 5 percent

Drinks

Balancing Food Proportions

The chart on page 17 is intended to give some idea of the proportions in which each food type can be used when preparing your menus for the day. It is to suit a temperate climate and does not have to be adhered to rigidly. Relax and enjoy preparing and varying your meals. Hundreds of different meals can be created—and created is the word!—by using different combinations.

Food categories may overlap. Soup to begin a meal might contain grains or beans, certainly sea vegetables or land vegetables and/or fish. Miso soup made from noodles with tofu can contain a little of everything and be a quick meal in itself. Vegetable courses may include salads and pickles when the weather is warmer. Try to use mainly vegetables, with animal products as an occasional supplement. It's not that you can't eat meat or anything else you wish, but once you get used to the clean, natural taste of vegetables and grains you will find meat rather heavy going. "Man is the prince of animals," said Ohsawa. "We have no need to feed ourselves with meat . . . too much meat protein (yang) results in thrombosis, cruelty and violence . . . vegetables are the supreme food, the normal, logical and pure source of food. Without vegetable life no animal on earth could survive. Our hemoglobin is derived

Barley

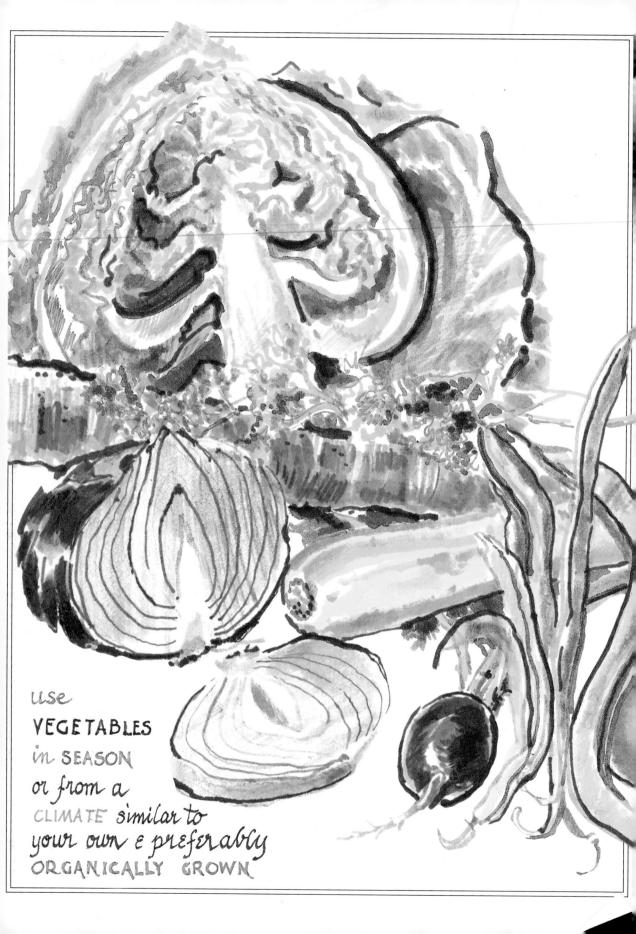

use
VEGETABLES
in SEASON
or from a
CLIMATE similar to
your own & preferably
ORGANICALLY GROWN

from chlorophyll." And he sums it all up with, "If it can protest or run away—don't eat it!"

Many factors will control the nature and content of your meal. You, the cook, will feel different each time you prepare food, as will your family or your friends. The weather will also be different and the seasonal vegetables available will give you new ideas about putting the ingredients together.

One thing is certain: If you cook calmly and with loving care, taking pleasure in the doing, it will be reflected in the results. Care is probably one of the most important ingredients of any meal.

Soup

Approximately 5 percent

Soup is an excellent start for a meal—it can also begin a day well for that matter. You should need no more than one or two cups or bowls of it each day. Good seasonings to use are tamari or miso.

For soup stock always keep the water after steaming or boiling vegetables. Improve it by bringing the water to a boil with some kombu in it. Other sea vegetables can be used, or bonito flakes—to give flavor and texture to soups (*see* INGREDIENTS—Sea Vegetables).

Miso soup can be a meal in itself with a selection of grains or noodles, beans or tofu, with land and sea vegetables. There are several different types of miso (*see* INGREDIENTS—Miso).

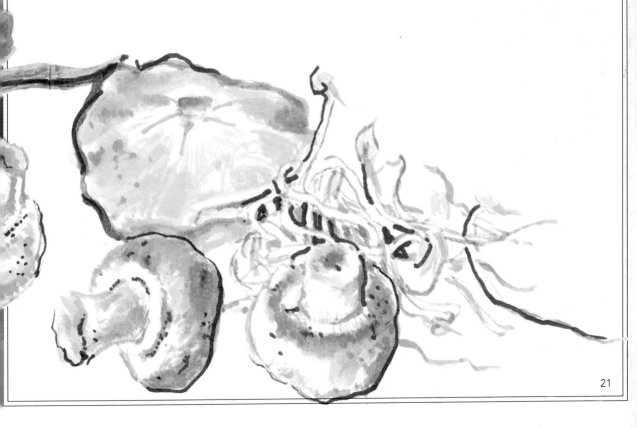

Grains, Your Principal Food

50 percent or more

The principal food—whole cereal grains and their products—should ideally make up 50 percent or more of your day's food and the volume of each meal.

Grains have served humankind for thousands of years and have been the principal food of practically every civilization. They need to remain humanity's primary food. The length of the human digestive tract is apparently more suited to dealing with grains and vegetables than with animal food.

But how modern humans abuse our grains! We refine them, we predigest them, we knock the life out of them and leave the polishings rich in nutrients to the livestock—who thrive! We then sell the refined grains in the supermarkets—poor, incomplete, unbalanced, and unnatural shadows of their former selves! No wonder they are not as popular as they used to be!

Get used to whole grains: They are alive and full of life energy, and they are a richer food than the cereal and flour products made from them. When grains are crushed or ground, they lose some of their vitality, especially if stored for any length of time. Flour products also tend to cause mucus in the body.

Chief Grains: Brown rice, millet, barley, whole wheat (bread, pastry, crackers and noodles), oats (oatmeal), maize or corn (cornmeal), buckwheat groats (noodles), rye (bread), and so forth (*see also* INGREDIENTS—Grains).

Legumes (Beans)

More or less 10 percent

Beans can be used as a side dish or can be mixed or cooked with your grain. They are useful for soups and spreads such as hummus made from chickpeas. There are a number of soybean ferment products such as tamari, tofu, and tempeh, which bring new flavors to a meal.

The serving of grains and beans together is important. The useable protein is increased considerably when the two are combined.

Beans blend well with sea vegetables. Cooking the beans with some seaweeds such as kombu strips or wakame helps to digest them. The sea minerals tend to balance the fat and protein of the beans.

Chief Beans: Aduki, chickpeas, lentils, black turtle and, for less frequent use, pinto, kidney beans, split peas (*see also* INGREDIENTS—Legumes).

Seeds

Seeds can be used sparingly as condiments. They should be washed, pan-roasted, or baked briefly, perhaps with a pinch of salt, or a few drops of soy sauce, but *no oil*—they already have a high oil content. They are tasty and crunchy sprinkled on grains, beans, or vegetables. Try roasted pumpkin seeds sprinkled over your freshly steamed kale. Roasted sesame seeds ground with a small amount of sea salt (gomasio) are often used. Sesame paste is used as a spread (*see* INGREDIENTS—Seeds).

Vegetables and Sea Vegetables

About 25 percent

VEGETABLES

Vegetables range from more modern land varieties down the evolutionary cycle to fungi, sea vegetables, and sea moss—all mainly cooked.

Land vegetables: The leaf and root varieties can be used in soups, can be served as separate side dishes or can be cooked with the main grain. They can be sautéed in water (or a little oil), steamed, boiled, baked, fried (using unrefined vegetable or seed oils). Some vegetables need only to be immersed briefly in boiling water. They can be served raw in warmer weather or as a lightly boiled salad, pressed salad, which is refreshing, or pickles.

Chief Vegetables: More modern species of temperate origin: carrot, burdock, parsnip, radish, daikon radish (mooli), salsify (and their leaves), cabbage, Chinese cabbage, lettuce, spinach, kale, parsley, watercress, arugula, Swiss chard, collard greens, mustard greens, cauliflower, celery, cucumber, squash, pumpkin, onion, leek, scallion (spring onion), green peas, string beans, dandelion, clover, bean sprouts, grain sprouts, etc.

More ancient or tropical species: potato, sweet potato, yam, tomato, eggplant, asparagus, green pepper, artichoke, bamboo shoot, okra, beets, lotus root, etc.

More primitive origin: mushroom and other fungi species.

In temperate climates it is not a good idea to use too many of the tropical species. Macrobiotics generally avoid potatoes, tomatoes, and eggplant. These are members of the *solanaceae,* or nightshade family, as are chili, cayenne pepper, tobacco, belladonna, and several other poisons and drugs.

SEA VEGETABLES

About a quarter of your vegetables can consist of sea varieties, which are a very special part of a macrobiotic meal. Incredibly rich in minerals, they can be served as a separate side dish, but they can also be combined with beans and are excellent for soups. Dulse and ulva are delicious in salads. Fresh Welsh laver (same family as nori) can be used as a spread or to make oatcakes.

Before cooking, most dried sea vegetables need only be immersed in water for a minute or two until soft. Soaking in water too long may extract minerals. Always use the same water for cooking the seaweed unless, as with some uncultivated species, deposits of sand or tiny shells remain after soaking.

Sea vegetables can also be roasted over a flame or in the oven, then ground to make condiments to flavor food. Agar-agar and carrageen make fine jellies (kanten), aspic, or jellied soup.

Chief Sea Vegetables: Agar-agar (kanten), arame, carrageen (Irish Moss), dulse, hijiki, kombu, laver, nori, wakame (*see* INGREDIENTS—Sea Vegetables).

Animal Products

5 percent or not more than 10 percent

If we choose to eat animal products—and in certain colder climates and polar regions humans need to do so—the less highly evolved species such as shellfish and fish are more suitable than are wild bird, chicken, and turkey, which in turn are preferable to meats like lamb, beef, and pork.

Once or twice a week then, but as a complementary side dish, *not* as a principal food, have some fish or shellfish. Faster moving, dark-meat fish are more yang than are slower-moving white-meat fish and shellfish varieties.

Nearly all cultivated animal products—chicken, pork, beef, butter, eggs, and milk are to some extent artificially produced and chemically treated. Wild, free-range birds are less likely to be so than domestic birds, and lamb is preferable to beef or pork for the same reason.

Always serve animal products with plenty of vegetables to balance the yang.

Chief Fish Species: Sole, halibut, hake, cod, salmon, trout, snapper, bluefish, whiting, flounder, haddock, smelt, carp, swordfish, tuna, shark, mackerel, sardine, anchovy, eel, and their roe.

Other Seafood: Oyster, clam, scallop, mussel, shrimp, lobster, crab.

Chief Amphibian Species: Frog, snail, turtle (and eggs).

Chief Bird Species: Chicken, turkey, duck, pheasant, partridge, and their eggs.

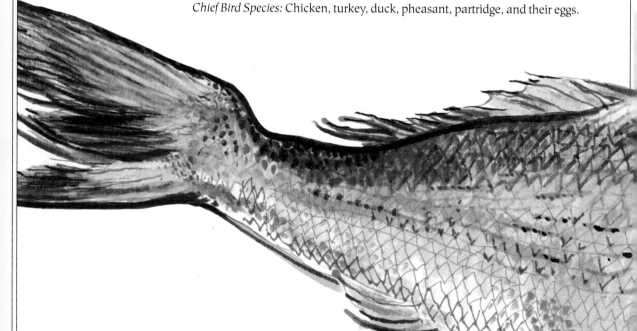

Chief Mammal Species: Rabbit, hare, boar, pig, goat, cattle, sheep, their milk and milk products.

Natural Enzymes and Bacteria: Enzymes are produced by the body during digestion. Fermented foods can be used to help this digestion process. The vegetable-based fermented foods are dealt with under the next section on condiments. Enzymes are also present in beer, whisky, wine, sake, and other fermented alcoholic drinks. Chief animal-fermented products are cheese, yogurt, and buttermilk.

Seasoning Your Food

Food should never taste salty. Use condiments only to bring out the natural flavors. When cooking in a temperate climate, the best seasoning to use is a pinch of *unrefined* sea salt or rock salt, which contains a correct balance of minerals invariably removed from "table" salt. Natural salt is an off-white color because of its mineral content. Refined salt is 99 percent sodium chloride; it is usually iodized and may even contain sugar to make it pour, or magnesium carbonate to bleach it white; phosphate of lime and other substances are often added.

There are several other vegetable-based fermented foods that are useful for seasoning. Tamari, soy sauce, miso and umeboshi plums are some of these. Each is to be used carefully.

Chief Condiments: sesame salt (gomasio), umeboshi plums, tekka, tamari, soy sauce, miso, roasted seaweed powder (*see* INGREDIENTS).

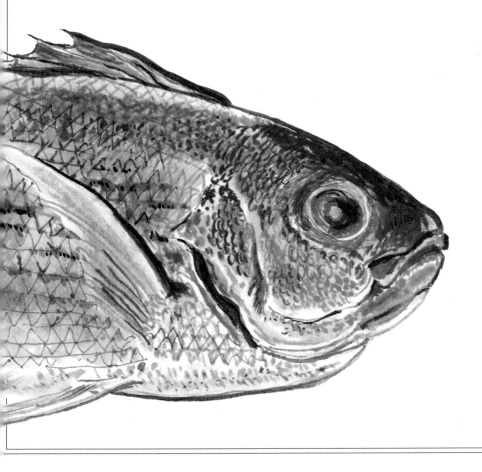

Desserts, Fruits and Nuts

A moderate 5 percent

Fruit needs to be used carefully even when in season. Fruit is the edible flesh around the seeds of plants and contains a great deal of sugar. Because of this we tend to devour it in large quantities. Apples, the most yang of fruits, are still much more yin than are vegetables and grains. They are delicious lightly cooked with agar-agar, to make kanten or jelly. Tropical fruits eaten in cold weather won't help keep you warm.

Natural desserts can be made by using more yang, sweet vegetables—pumpkin or squash pie for example. Sweet brown rice, aduki beans, and chestnuts can also be used. Dried fruits and raisins are useful for sweetening or sweeten with small quantities of barley malt or rice syrup.

Grain products and beans can be used to make rice cakes, puddings, popcorn, pastry, cereals, and cookies or crackers.

Chief Temperate Zone Fruits: Apples, cherries, peaches, plums, apricots, strawberries, blueberries, blackberries, raspberries, cantaloupe and various local melons, watermelon, pears, peaches, grapes, mandarin oranges.

Chief Tropical Fruits: Oranges, lemons, limes, pineapple, coconut, mango, papaya, banana, avocado.

Chief Nuts: Almonds, walnuts, hazelnuts, chestnuts, pine nuts, cashews, peanuts. The more oily nuts are Brazil nuts and pecans (*see* INGREDIENTS—Nuts).

A few roasted ground or whole nuts are delicious served over desserts, cooked in cakes or biscuits and added to muesli. Like seeds, nuts taste much better fresh from the shell and roasted. Use sea salt or a little tamari to season them from time to time. Don't use oil as they have a high oil content. Nut butters such as peanut butter should be used sparingly. Sesame seed paste (tahini) is preferred, but it also has a high oil content.

What to Drink

Cooked grains and vegetables contain a great deal of water, which reduces the need for drinking too much extra liquid.

Try not to drink with your meal—it dilutes the digestive juices, which can cause trouble. Beverages may be taken during the last part of the meal, with dessert, or alone when needed.

I think one of the turning points in my drinking career was a moment during a rehearsal break when I found myself throwing several large spoons of white sugar into a cup of the BBC's finest rehearsal-brewed coffee—just to make it palatable. That bitter, milky, chemical taste just wasn't good enough—and it was hard to disguise!

There are no chemical additives in macrobiotic teas or coffees. They are made from herbs and roasted roots, and once you are used to the flavor of nature you will wonder how you could ever have put up with anything else.

Bancha and *Kukicha (twig tea)* (*see* INGREDIENTS—Teas) are the most refreshing drinks for all occasions. They taste very much like "ordinary" or what some call "normal" tea but, being free of additives, they taste cleaner—and do you more good. *Green tea* is more bitter (*see* INGREDIENTS—

Teas). *Dandelion* and *burdock roots* and grains can make excellent coffees or teas when roasted. *Mint tea* is not used too often, but it is a good digestive and is a refreshing summer drink. *Chamomile tea* is good for the vocal chords—by inhaling the steam or as a gargle. *Mu tea* is a combination of herbs and is delicious served with a dash of apple juice (*see* INGREDIENTS—Teas).

Apple juice should be the main summer fruit juice used. Make sure it has no additives. Apples are a fruit local to most temperate climates. Juices are, however, only part of the whole fruit and even sweeter!

Still mineral water with a squeeze of fresh lemon juice is a drink for very hot weather. A slice of lemon in boiling water is fine for breakfast. Needless to say, carbonated drinks and alcohol are not encouraged! Ohsawa apparently enjoyed his drop of whisky. In fact, different macrobiotic books suggest different alcoholic beverages. They seem to vary according to the preference of the author! Some suggest a good-quality beer or cider, while others advocate sake, and Ohsawa ordered his whisky neat—they *are*, after all, mainly grain products! Michio Kushi advises that "small amounts of fermented or alcoholic beverages may be taken b*efore* the meal if the first part is soup . . . to smooth the appetite and digestion!"

Chief Beverages: Bancha tea, twig tea *(kukicha),* maté tea, green tea, mu (herb) tea, dandelion tea or coffee, burdock tea, comfrey tea, unsweetened grain coffee, roasted barley tea *(mugicha),* rice or other grain teas, and other traditional nonaromatic teas.

Fermented Alcoholic Beverages: Beer, cider, sake, whisky, wine.

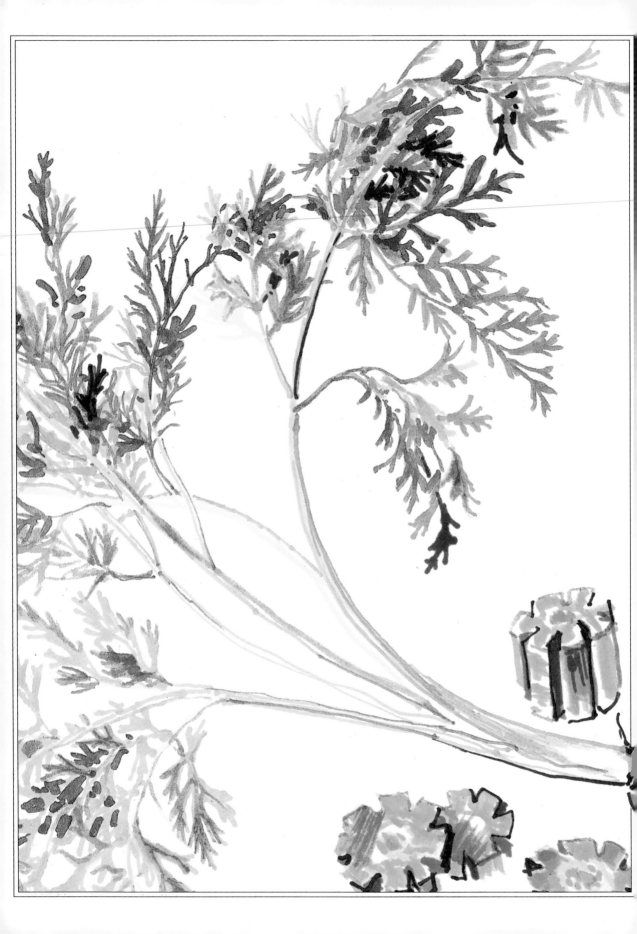

Any Questions Before Cooking?

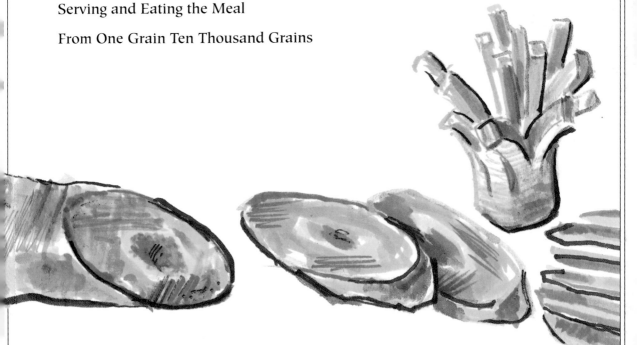

Why Organic Foods?

Vegetables grown organically are sometimes difficult to find in big cities. Such vegetables can cost more, too, if they aren't covered with insecticides—"artificial protection science misguidedly offers us"—but if the insects won't eat these products, why should we?

Some people say you can't tell the difference between an organically and a chemically grown product, but you generally can. The larger, more colorful and shinier the fruit, the more likely it is to be puffed up with fertilizers or sprayed with hormone mixtures. It may look appealing on the supermarket shelves, but the natural flavor will almost certainly be missing. Smaller fruits and vegetables are more yang—Ohsawa says that a small red apple has a lower potassium-sodium ratio than a large green one. Those highly colored carrots (probably dyed!), straight and clean (probably grown in fertilized sand), and probably waxed (to make them shine) will have to be scraped thoroughly. If they are crooked shapes, are somewhat dusty with tops attached (valuable greens—use them!) they are probably organic as advertised and only need a rinse or gentle scrub with your bristle brush before cooking.

Why Fruits and Vegetables in Season?

(Or from a similar climate?)

Tropical fruits and vegetables are fine when eaten where the sun blazes down, but in the depths of an English winter or a New York snowstorm they can make us feel cold. They are more yin, designed by nature to balance the yang, hot weather conditions in which they grew. Eating them continually—and people who come from tropical climates to live in colder places tend to do so—can cause a great deal of unhappiness and sickness. Imported foods also need to be treated with preservatives in order to travel. Fruits and vegetables are allowed by law to be washed with retarding agents, to be treated with antisprouting agents or with enzyme inhibitors to prevent further growth.

Fruit juices come under this category. They are generally synthetic anyway, with chemical flavorings to delight the palate. Even real, fresh orange juice may be all right for a Spanish or Moroccan summer or a Florida beach (in moderation!) but should not become a daily habit. Pure apple juice, made from organically grown apples, is a better fruit drink for summer—but check the labels for additives and use it moderately. Remember, there are quite a few parts of the fruit missing from the juice.

Why Whole Foods?

There are huge vested interests in converting natural whole foods into precooked, processed food in order to make your life simpler in the kitchen and to control the shelf life of the product. During processing, however, literally thousands of chemicals, drugs, preservatives, stabilizers, softeners, sweeteners, alkalizers, acidifiers, emulsifiers, hormones, dyes, antioxidants and hydrogenants all find their way into our diets without our realizing it. According to the London Food Commission Report, autumn 1985, two thousand tons of additives are now used each year by British manufacturers alone—over eight pounds annually per consumer! Dietary diseases resulting, it claims, from our consumption of so much processed starch, fat, and sugar, cost the National Health Service over £1 billion a year. They will go on doing so unless we consumers do something about it! Such foods include those brightly colored bottles of soda, soft and iced drinks, sugared sweets, saccharine syrups, all artificially flavored, those potato chips, candy, and incandescent popsicles we ply our kids with to please them. ("They might as well eat their school chemistry set," the above Food News report dryly observes.) The TV commercials for all these products are lavish because the manufacturers are very rich.

The food value of such products is, on the other hand, usually very poor. Perhaps one of the most serious causes of deprivation in our affluent society is the removal of vital nutrients from our chief food sources: bread, flour, and grains. White bread, white flour, white rice, and, the worst of all, white sugar! Ohsawa said that the harmfulness of white sugar is much more terrible than is imagined. Try to avoid sugar and sugar products. The natural sugar content of fruits and vegetables is really sweetness enough (*see* THE BODY—A LABORATORY, Vitamins, Carbohydrates, Sugar).

Why Less Animal Products?

There is a seventeenth-century English proverb, "Much meat, much maladies," and today's nutritionists are practically unanimous about the effects of eating too much meat. It does contain protein, but fish or grains with beans can contain as much, if not more. Michio Kushi suggests that of the thirty teeth in our head twenty of them are premolars suitable for grinding grains and cereals, eight are incisors for cutting vegetables and four are canines for tearing at food. He thus arrives at the proportion of twenty-eight teeth for vegetables to four for meat—his golden ratio of 7:1! While strict vegetarians may need to watch their vitamin B_6 and B_{12} supply, meat eaters need to exercise their own form of caution: Nearly all cultivated animals or their produce—chicken, pork, beef, butter, eggs, and milk—are chemically treated at some stage. If you ever go in a shed full of caged, drugged chickens with their beaks cut, you will wonder about the quality of the meat and eggs being mass-produced there for you. The recent "Mad Cow" epidemics were caused by introducing slaughterhouse waste into the diet of vegetarian animals. This gives cause for great concern.

"Animal milk," said Ohsawa, "is the ideal composition for an animal unaccustomed to thinking . . . cow's milk is, after all, intended to be nourishment for calves!" Milk intake is now being associated with some alarming diseases. Meat, milk, and eggs are high in cholesterol and saturated fats (*see* THE BODY—A LABORATORY, Protein, Calcium, and Saturated Fats).

Which Pots and Pans?

One nutritionist writes, "Copper can neutralize and aluminum poison your vitamin supply." Macrobiotic cooks Wendy and Edward Esko recommend heavy *cast iron pans* and *skillets*. The latter are certainly extremely useful, but a strong right arm is sometimes needed to handle the larger ones. They do distribute the heat evenly, but there is a remote possibility that too much iron may be served with the food if iron pots are used exclusively (*see* THE BODY—A LABORATORY, Trace Elements, Iron).

Ceramic pots are excellent for cooking grains and beans. They need a flame deflector or cast iron stand to prevent strong direct heat, and sudden temperature changes can crack them. Any pan needs to be left to cool before pouring cold water over it. Even cast iron will suffer from this treatment.

Stainless-steel pots, especially with reinforced heavy bottoms, are practical. Use lower heat, though, as they absorb heat directly and can burn the food. A *stainless-steel pressure cooker* is usually recommended: They save fuel and cook food quickly. Pressure yangizes the food, too.

Pyrex pots and ovenware are more fragile, but they are light, clean, and easy to handle. You can see what is going on while the food is cooking.

Enameled iron pots are useful, but they do chip, and the enamel scratches if metal or steel wool pads are used to clean them.

What Other Utensils?

There are several other items you can buy for the kitchen. Some you will own already if you enjoy cooking.

Wooden spoons and ladles won't scratch your pans and are kind to the food.

A *natural bristle brush* is ideal for gently scrubbing your root vegetables under water.

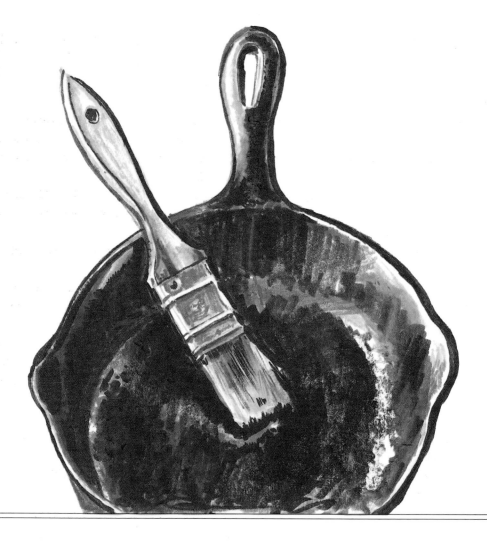

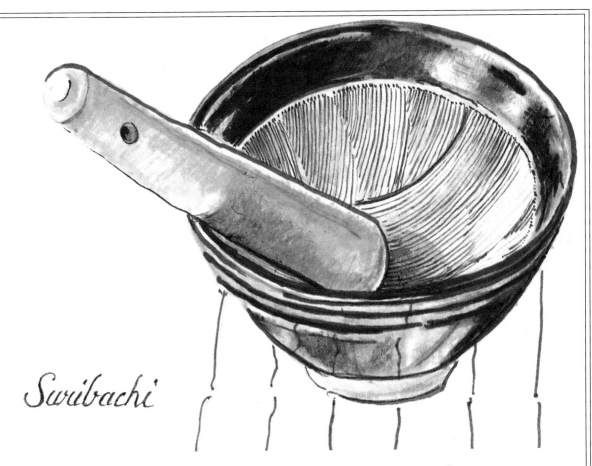

Suribachi

A *good vegetable knife* with a carbon steel blade is probably the best investment. It cuts cleanly and helps you make attractive patterns of your vegetables to decorate a meal. You will need a whetstone, which is quite therapeutic to use. The carbon steel blade needs sharpening only along one side of the cutting edge. Stainless steel blades are fine, but they can chip.

A *wooden chopping block*—a good-sized one—for your vegetable cutting is a must. Oil it with sesame oil from time to time and try not to wash it with soap. Just wipe it with a wet cloth before starting and between each differently flavored vegetable.

Glass or ceramic jars, or even wooden ones, are useful for storing your grains, beans, and nuts. Make sure the tops are an airtight fit.

A *grinding bowl or suribachi,* with a wooden pestle is useful for grinding your sesame salt, mixing your miso thoroughly, making salad dressings, creams, pureeing food for babies, etc. This process is gentler than using a noisy electric blender. Less washing up too!

A *Sushi mat* is a small, flexible mat made from fine strips of bamboo that are strung together. It is so called because it is used to make sushi rolls (*see* Sushi), but it has a number of other functions in the kitchen. It can cover food while it cools, it can keep it warm, or it can even be used as a table mat to protect table surfaces from hot pans (*see* page 157).

A *bamboo strainer* is available to strain your bancha or twig tea.

A *stainless-steel steamer* is one of the best cooking instruments for vegetables. After a minute or two, greens turn a vibrant, chlorophyll color, which means they're ready to be eaten.

A *grater.* A flat one for general use is the most practical. There are also some attractive china ones for grating ginger that are now available.

33

Preparing Vegetables

Vegetables need to be kept fresh until the moment you cook them. First wash them carefully—roots need a gentle scrub—but soaking them for hours in gallons of water destroys their vital nutrients.

Cutting vegetables can add to their appearance and help balance their yin-yang quality. That sharp knife is needed, but be careful of your fingers! Keep them out of harm's way by curling them under at the first knuckle of the fingers holding the vegetable. Place the side of the blade against your knuckle and the front end of the cutting edge gently on the vegetable and thrust smoothly away from you the full length of the blade. Try not to saw backward and forward or to treat the vegetables too roughly. Roots are usually sliced on the diagonal, and vegetables such as onion, for example, from top to bottom rather than across to include as much of their yin-yang property in each portion as possible. The top of a root is more yin than is the base. There are several patterns you can make—triangular, half-moon, diced, matchsticks, chrysanthemums, rectangles, quarters, and flowers. Roots such as carrots and burdock also can be shaved as you would sharpen a pencil or rolled as you cut them. Keep the pieces small.

It has been said before and no doubt will be said again—never use too much water for cooking vegetables and save it for soup, stock, and sauces. Most leaf vegetables need only to be boiled briefly in a little water or steamed for a minute or so and they are ready. It's a good idea to plunge vegetables quickly into boiling water to seal them and protect water-soluble vitamins as much as possible.

Never use too much oil when sautéing either. You generally need only brush the pan or skillet with oil and use low heat. Avoid commercial cooking oils, rendered fats, lards, margarine, etc. Sesame, corn, soy, sunflower, safflower, and sometimes olive oils are the best to use. Make sure they are cold pressed or unrefined. Extracted oils have usually been subjected to high temperatures, which changes the quality of the oil. Heating your pan until the oil smokes can mean a loss of vitamin E (*see* THE BODY—A LABORA-TORY, Fats. *For deep-frying see* INGREDIENTS—Oils, Tempura).

Serving and Eating the Meal

Having prepared your meal with care, be careful now not to pile the plates high with mounds of grains or to fill the bowls to the brim: large portions can be daunting. "Sometimes," said Ohsawa, "when confronted by an Occidental vegetarian meal I feel as sad as if I had been turned into a horse because of the coarse consistency of the food. . . . The quantity of the food changes the quality," he said. "You can have too much even of a good thing." Ohsawa took the view that every disease is caused by excess in diet, and he claimed he never saw one patient who was suffering from lack of food. Grains in particular can look and taste unappetizing if not served well. They generally need a sauce of some kind. Always prepare *and* present the food with an awareness of the yin-yang balance of textures, tastes, and colors.

Before eating the meal you have prepared—or that has been prepared for you—give yourself a moment's calm to think and to be grateful. Don't rush at it.

Gandhi said, "Chew your drink and drink your food." Chew each mouthful of food at least thirty times. Ohsawa suggests fifty—even a hundred or more—as stress on the jaws might help curb excess indulgence! This makes good sense, as saliva lubricates and begins breaking down our food before it is swallowed, and the pressure of chewing is also yang. Chewing helps calm your body as the miracle of digestion begins.

From One Grain Ten Thousand Grains

I was staying in a luxurious hotel on film location for a few weeks where the chef kindly cooked some brown rice. The waiter, when asked for a second helping, explained it had already been thrown out. "Everything," he said, "*had* to be."

This brought home the incredible waste of food that must take place daily in hotels and restaurants all over the world. I thought of the macrobiotic maxim, a small voice in a big world, *"From one grain ten thousand grains."* If everyone in the world threw away just one grain of rice we would lose enough grains to feed a million, and from each of these grains might grow ten thousand to feed some billion more.

My arithmetic isn't all that good, but the maxim brings with it a sharp reminder of how precious food is. Prepare natural food carefully, eat it with gratitude, and appreciate it to the last grain.

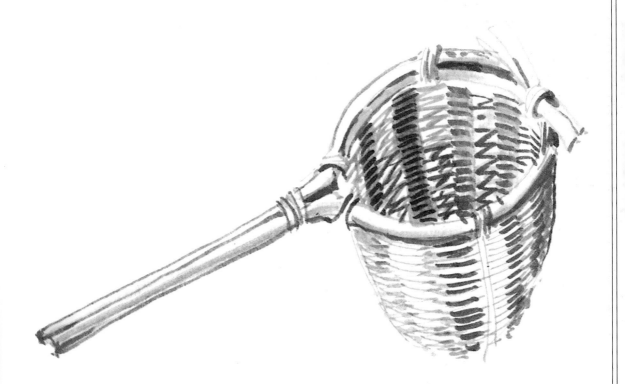

Bamboo tea strainer

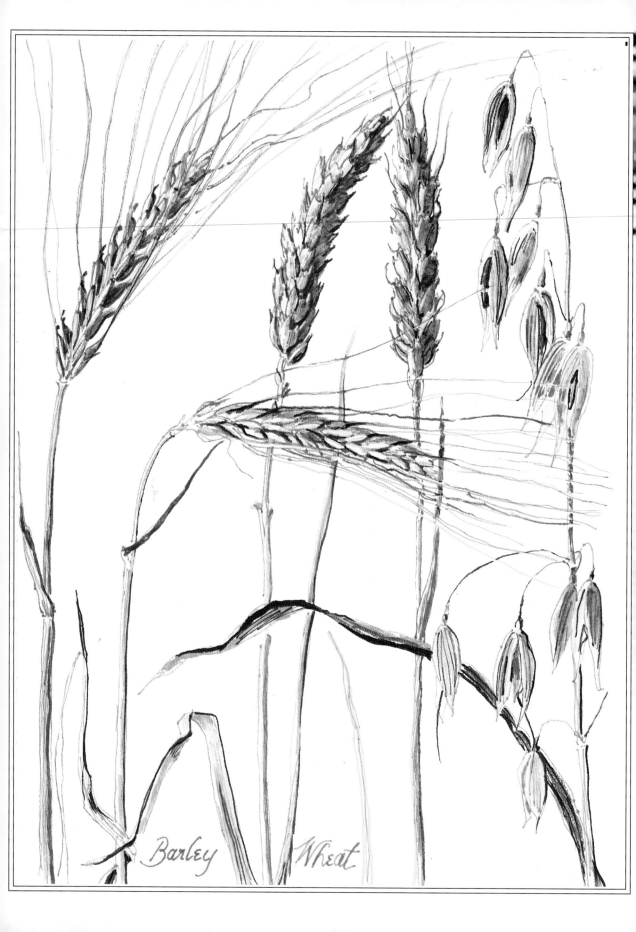

Barley Wheat

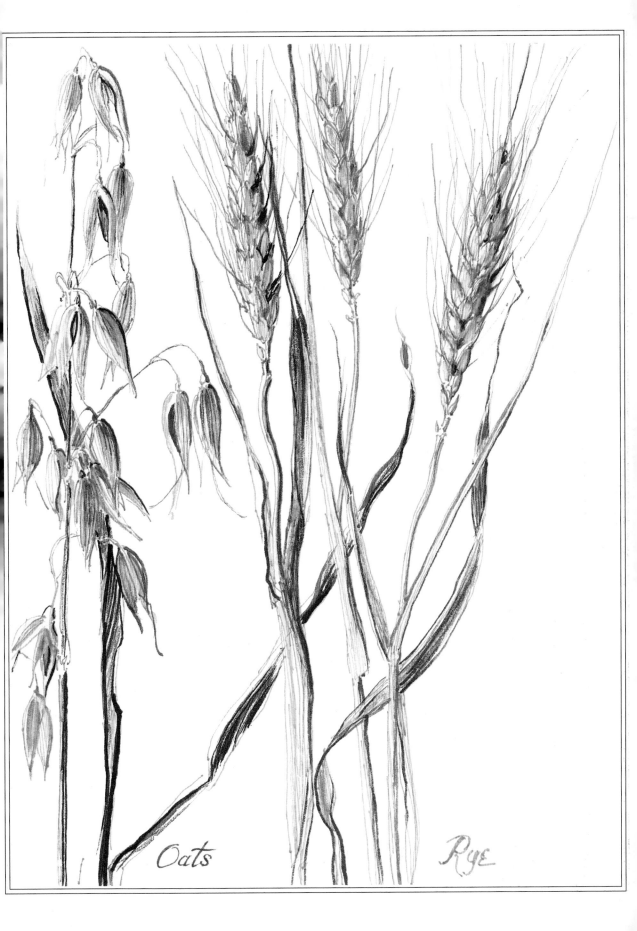

Oats

Rye

Ingredients

The names of some of these new, natural ingredients may sound strange to you, but don't be discouraged! They have been introduced from different parts of the world and from different cultures—some from the Orient, some from the Middle East, Europe, and Russia; the Welsh and the Irish still use sea vegetables, and the Scots know their oats—or did before oats were refined and packaged! Properly prepared, these new supplies are a real food source and have been used as such for centuries in their places of origin. Most traditional dishes were in fact originally well balanced—and practically macrobiotic!

The better cook you are the more fun you are going to have experimenting with the new ingredients, and the better your cooking will be because the quality of your raw materials will be vastly improved. The difference it can make to the texture, flavor—and benefit—of your meals is unbelievable.

About the Food Content Lists

Calculations from different samples of the same food can vary considerably. This is because factors such as the soil in which the food was grown, the season, the variety of plant, growing conditions, and so forth, all vary, as does the length of time the food is stored and handled. Vitamin figures for foods containing water (for example, some fruits and vegetables) can also be inconsistent since water is the most variable component. The list will, though, give some idea of which foods are nutrient sources. Values are usually for uncooked food.

The food content lists are averages of different food samples and the absence of a particular nutrient (–) does not necessarily mean that it is not in that particular food but that reliable information may not be available. (*See* Food Content information following each ingredient)

The quantities are usually measured in milligrams per 100 grams (4 ounces) of food in micrograms, or in the case of vitamins A and D in International Units. To give an idea of how small these weights are, 1 milligram is 1/1000th part of a gram (or 0.000035 of an ounce!). A microgram is 1/1000th of that!

REFERENCES

Macrobiotic Home Remedies by Michio Kushi; *Nutrition Almanac* by John D. Kirschmann, Nutrition Search, Inc., *Nutrition for a Better Life* by Nan Bronfen; *Introducing Macrobiotic Cooking* by Wendy Esko; *Macrobiotic Cooking for Everyone* by Edward and Wendy Esko; *The Natural Food Catalogue* by Vicki Peterson; *The Book of Tofu* by Shurtleff and Aoyagi; *The Book of Miso* by Shurtleff and Aoyagi; *The Book of Tempeh* by Shurtleff and Aoyagi; *Vegetables from the Sea* by S. and T. Araskai; *Cooks*

Ingredients by Davell and Bailey; *Composition and Facts About Food* by Ford Heritage; *Sushi* by Mi Detrick; *Whole Meals* by Marcea Weber; *The Truth About Bancha Tea* by Leonard Jacobs, East West Journal; *Standard Tables of Food Composition in Japan*, 1982, Ridal Press testing facilities; *The Structure of Everyday Life* by Fernand Brandel.

Agar-Agar

(*See* Sea Vegetables and Kanten.)

Amazake

Amazake is a sweet rice ferment sold as a drink now. It has the texture of milk because it is blended and strained and can be used to make jellies and creams. Unblended, it has the texture of rice pudding and is, in fact, delicious as such.

Here is a recipe for homemade amazake.

> 1 cup cooked brown rice (*see* Grains)
> 4 cups water
> 1 cup sweet brown rice (koji)
> Pinch of salt
> 1 cup warm water

1. Mix the koji and rice in a glass or ceramic bowl with a pinch of salt, and add the warm water (1 cup) to keep the mixture from sticking to the pan.
2. Cover the pot and incubate at body temperature (98°) for 6 to 8 hours, either by leaving on a "low" electric plate or covered in a very low oven or even in a warm cupboard.
3. After it has incubated, the amazake should taste sweet. Bring to a boil (add a little more water if necessary, but only to keep it from sticking). Boil for 5 to 10 minutes.
4. Let cool. Refrigerate in a glass bowl or jar.

Amazake can be used to make rice pudding by adding a teaspoon of lemon peel, 1/2 teaspoon cinnamon, and 1/2 cup raisins. It will serve 6 to 8. It can also be blended if a smoother texture is desired (*see also* Koji).

Aduki Beans *(Azuki)*

(*See* Legumes.)

Barley Malt

Barley malt is a sweetener or grain honey made from sprouting barley that is cooked into a sweet syrup. Nothing else is added: The barley is steeped in water to soften it, is germinated, and then heat is applied to dry the malt and bring out the flavor. A syrup is produced, which has the consistency of maple syrup, contains dextrins, maltose, dextrose, minerals, and protein.

Because it is less sweet than either honey or maple syrup, you may be tempted to use too much when cooking. (*See also* THE BODY—A LABORATORY, Chemistry of Carbohydrates.)

Food Content of Barley Malt (per 100 g): calories, 295; protein, 3.5 g; carbohydrate, 67.5 g; calcium, 80 mg; phosphorus, (–); iron, 2.0 mg; sodium, (–); potassium, (–); vitamin B_1, 0.04 mg; vitamin B_2, 0.035 mg; niacin, 4 mg; vitamin C, 8 mg. (Source: USDA)

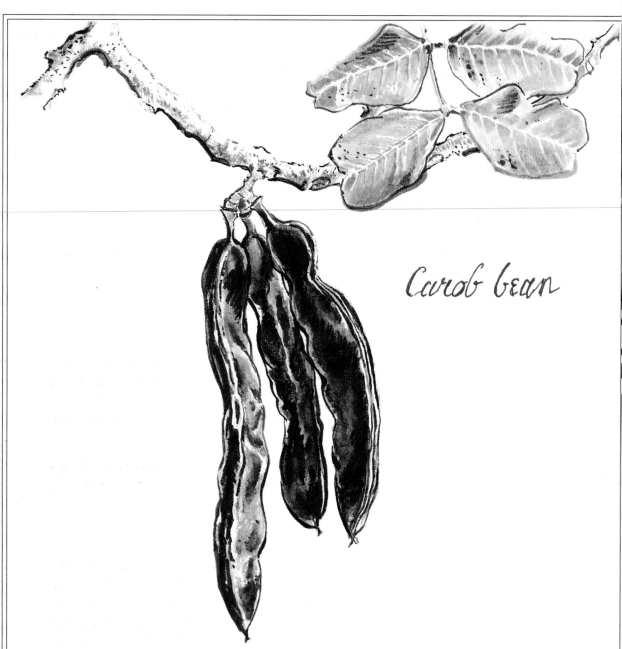

Carob bean

Bonito Flakes

Paper-thin flakes shaved from the dried fermented bonito fish *(hanakatsuo)* are used for soup stocks or to garnish soups or noodles.

Brown Rice

(See Grains.)

Brown Rice Vinegar

This is vinegar made from fermented brown rice in agricultural communities of Japan. Organic brown rice is used with a white rice *koji,* seed vinegar from the previous year and well water. The fermentation takes nine or ten months. Brown rice vinegar is sharp in flavor and is useful for salads and for keeping vegetables fresh. It is good sprinkled over grated daikon radish, on a sea vegetable, or pressed salad. A salad dressing can also be made by mixing it with apple juice or lemon juice and a little olive or sesame oil. It will also add piquancy to sauces.

Buckwheat or Kasha

(See Grains.)

Burdock Root *(Artium lappa)*

This wild, hardy, thistlelike plant is common to the Northern Hemisphere—England, northern Europe, and the United States. The Japanese name for it is *gobo* and the entire plant—young leaf, stems, and the root—can be used. The leaves for salad and greens and the root will give your cooking a rich, earthy flavor. According to herbalists the long, black root is one of the finest blood purifiers, and is of benefit to rheumatism sufferers; used externally, it will help skin ailments. It is even claimed to be a sexual restorative in the Orient. It is certainly one of the most yang roots.

Before cooking, burdock root will need washing and a gentle scrub. Slice it diagonally or in matchsticks or whatever pattern you decide, then soak the sections in water for ten to fifteen minutes (the water will go green). Burdock needs to be cooked longer than do most root vegetables. It can also be purchased as an unusual and invigorating herbal tea. Boil the dried, dark chips in water (1 teaspoon per cup) for 5 to 10 minutes.

Food Content of Burdock (per 100 g): calories, 75; protein, 4.1 g; fat, 0.1 g; carbohydrate 16.3 g; calcium, 47 mg; phosphorus, 71 mg; iron, 0.8 mg; sodium, 45 mg; potassium, (–); vitamin B_1, 0.03 mg; vitamin B_2, 0.05 mg; 4 mg; vitamin C, 2 mg.

Carob *(St. John's Bread)*

Carob is a legume or bean and belongs to the locust family. The edible pods and beans from this tall, green, shady tree have been a source of food for thousands of years for humans and animals. When St. John the Baptist lived in the wilderness on locusts and wild honey it was the dark, purple carob or locust bean—not the insect—he was enjoying! And a very "yin" diet it would seem to be! The use of carob is increasingly recommended in place of chocolate, which contains caffeine and needs to be artificially sweetened—usually with white sugar—while carob does not. Carob flour is regarded as interchangeable with chocolate powder and is a good substitute for it in cooking cakes and desserts.

Food Content of Carob (per 100 g): calories, 175; protein, 50 g; fat, 1.25 g; carbohydrate, 81.3 g; fiber, 8 g; calcium, 350 mg; phosphorus, 75 mg; iron, 4.25 mg; sodium, (–); potassium, (–).

Daikon or Mooli

This long, white radish root is sold by many greengrocers now and is used by Chinese cooks. It makes a delicious side dish or a salad served grated with a few drops of tamari or umeboshi vinegar. It also makes a refreshing pressed salad (grated with carrot and cucumber, sprinkled with a couple pinches of salt, then pressed for 45 minutes), or it can be cooked in soups or stews. It is good for the digestion of oily foods and is said to "cut" fat and mucous deposits in the body.

Daikon greens are also a rich food source. Boil them quickly as green vegetables, or steam them.

Food Content of Daikon (per 100 g): [greens in brackets] calories, 19 [49]; protein, 0.9 g [5.2 g]; fat, 0.1 g [0.7 g] carbohydrate, 4.2 g [8.5 g]; fiber, 0.7 g [1.4 g]; calcium, 35 mg [190 mg]; phosphorus, 26 mg [30 mg]; iron, 0.6 mg [1.4 mg]; sodium, (–) [100 mg]; potassium, 180 mg [–]; vitamin A, 10 IU [3,000 IU]; vitamin B$_1$, 0.03 mg [0.1 mg]; vitamin B$_2$, 0.02 mg [0.3 mg]; vitamin B$_3$, 0.4 mg [0.5 mg]; vitamin C, 32 mg [90 mg].

Dashi

Probably the most important ingredient of noodle dishes is the broth in which they are served. Here is a recipe for "dashi," which is a clear soup made as follows:

8 cups water
2 pinches kombu powder (see SEA VEGETABLES)
2 teaspoons bonito flakes
1/3 cup soaked wakame or 6 shiitake mushrooms
3/4 cup soaking water
2 tablespoons tamari
2 tablespoons mirin or sake (optional) or 1 teaspoon barley malt

1. Place kombu in water and bring to a boil.
2. Slice wakame into small squares (chop ribs very fine). Add wakame (with soaking water) or bonito flakes and simmer for 10 minutes.
3. Soak mushrooms for 15 minutes in water. Remove stalk ends and slice finely. Add mushrooms and soaking water to kombu and bonito flakes.
4. Simmer for 20 minutes. Add tamari and mirin or sake or barley malt. Serve with noodles.

Serves 4 to 6

Denti

This is black tooth powder made of sea salt and charred eggplant (aubergine). The powder is used as a gargle before brushing the teeth. It will also stop bleeding if applied to cuts.

Dulse

(*See* Sea Vegetables.)

Ginger

Ginger is a golden-colored, pungent, spicy root vegetable with a multitude of uses as a condiment in cooking. This tropical plant is now grown in many hot countries such as Australia. Because of its shape the root is called "hand" or "finger" and is said to have medicinal properties. A compress made with grated ginger and very hot water will stimulate circulation and "dissolve stagnation," which can help kidney problems, stomach aches, and intestinal problems such as constipation and diarrhea (*not* appendicitis), stiffness of shoulders and joints, sinus troubles, cysts, and neuralgia—even toothache.

Here is a recipe for making a ginger compress:

> 8 cups water
> 3 tablespoons grated, fresh ginger
> 1 piece cheesecloth, 6 inches square

1. Bring water *almost* to a boil and remove from heat.
2. Tie the cheesecloth around the grated ginger and drop it into the hot water.
3. Let the ginger stew, covered, for 10 minutes. The water will become milky.
4. Squeeze the juice from the cheesecloth and remove it from the hot water.
5. To apply a compress, roll up a cotton towel or cloth. Hold each end and dip the center into the hot ginger water. Keeping the ends dry will enable you to wring out excess water without burning your fingers.

Place the hot compress over the affected area. It should be as hot as you can stand it. Cover with a thick, dry towel to keep in the heat. When the compress has cooled (5 minutes or so), reheat ginger water and repeat the process several times until the skin becomes red.

Food Content of Fresh Root Ginger (per 100 g): calories, 49; protein, 1.4 g; fat, 1.0 g; carbohydrate, 9.5 g; fiber, 1.1 g; calcium, 23 mg; phosphorus, 36 mg; iron, 2.1 mg; sodium, 6 mg; potassium, 264 mg; vitamin A, 10 IU; vitamin B$_1$, 0.20 mg; vitamin B$_2$, 0.04 mg; vitamin B$_3$, 0.7 mg; vitamin C, 4 mg.

Gomasio *(Sesame Salt)*

Gomasio is a popular condiment made from sesame seeds and sea salt. Prepare it as follows:

> 15 to 20 teaspoons sesame seeds
> 1 teaspoon sea salt or rock salt

1. Dry roast the seeds in a skillet to a golden brown. Stir well to prevent burning.
2. Place seeds with salt in your suribachi and grind well to make a fragrant-smelling condiment. You can use the coffee grinder to blend, but take care—you could end up with butter instead!

Gomasio, or sesame salt, sprinkled over your rice and vegetables, salads or cereal in the morning gives them a delicate nutty flavor. Use it sparingly, and don't make too much at a time. Renew your supply every few days and keep it stored in an airtight container in a cool, dark place. Although the salt helps preserve the crushed seeds, they still deteriorate and the flavor is better if made fresh. Ohsawa claimed that children who are fretful and cry too much are helped by a teaspoon of this condiment sprinkled over their food each day. It is also said to help certain types of headache.

(*See also* Seeds—Sesame.)

Grains

Grains are the edible fruit seeds of cereal grasses. To many people they are synonymous with animal fodder, but in fact whole grains have been the staple food of all major civilizations. However, particularly over the past thirty or forty years, there has been a drastic increase in commercial processing. Nutrients are extracted from grains, depleting our supply and upsetting the natural fundamental balance in our diet, depriving us of a rich source of vitamins and minerals. Refined grains are generally pretty tasteless, far less satisfying to eat, and certainly less nourishing. The insecticides, additives, bleaches, and dyes used on them in the various modern processes haven't improved them either!

The rediscovery of the whole and vital grain is perhaps the most exciting aspect of macrobiotics; certainly no meal seems complete without them. However, you need to learn to cook them well and serve them with some seasoning, vegetables, or sauce. A woman came to my dressing room one night complaining that she'd tried "my" brown rice. She had, she confessed, only cooked it for fifteen minutes! Whole grains do take rather longer to cook than the processed, precooked stuff—put them on while you prepare the rest of the meal. Grains are better eaten whole than as flakes or flours. Even the simple process of milling grain can destroy the natural balance and many of the nutrients it contains. The whole grains also last longer. They should be kept in airtight containers in a cool, dark place. Flours, on the other hand, need to be used as soon as possible. For this reason hand grinding mills are becoming popular. The flour can be made when needed.

There are several types of grains and many delicious ways to prepare them as the main course of your meal.

BARLEY *(Hordium vulgare)*

Barley is believed to be the oldest cultivated grain. It is a relation of the rice plant and a native of Mesopotamia, where it was used to make breads and was fermented to make beer. There are traces of barley cultivation at Neolithic sites dated 8000 B.C. in the Middle East, and there are numerous references to it in the Bible. Ancient settlements in Egypt (4500 B.C.) and Switzerland (3000 B.C.) show how long it has been used by humankind. In the Sumerian civilization, from around 4000 B.C., it was used as monetary currency—so many sacks for a day's work. By the Middle Ages in Europe, it was chiefly replaced by wheat and rye, but as barley is an adaptable grain that grows in different climates, it is still the staple food of many countries in the Far East, Asia, Middle East, and parts of Europe and South America. The people of Tibet consider it their most important food. In North America it is used mainly to make beer and alcoholic drinks or to feed livestock. In Scotland it is still used today for cooking the classic Scotch broths, and malted barley is used to make whisky, gin, and beer. In Japan barley is called *mugi* and a tea made by roasting the grains and then boiling them in water is called *mugicha*. There is also a delicious *mugi* miso. Barley is a delicious food that is high in nutrients and lower in fat than most other grains. When combined with rice or other grains it makes them much lighter in texture. Pot or Scotch barley is less refined than is light, pearled barley, which is the partially polished berry. Barley is delicious in soups, of course, or in vegetable-grain dishes, pies, or stuffings. You can roast the grains and grind them into flour to make bread or pastries.

To cook barley:

>   1 cup barley
>   4 to 5 cups water
>   Pinch of ground kombu (or sea salt)

1. Wash the grains and soak overnight—some cooks soak barley for two days.
2. Place grains in pot and add a cup of water and kombu or sea salt. Bring to a boil.
3. Turn down heat, cover, and simmer gently for 11/2 hours. Add more water if necessary.
4. Serve hot, garnished with chopped scallions or parsley and gomasio or tahini sauce.
Barley can be roasted before cooking for a change of flavor. It will then cook a little faster.

Food Content of Barley (pearled) (per 100 g): calories, carbohydrate, 79.0 g; 349; fiber, 0.4 g; fat, 1.4 g; protein, 8.2 g; calcium, 16 mg; phosphorus, 189 mg; sodium, potassium, 160 mg; 3 mg; iron, 2.0 mg; sulfur, 240 mg; magnesium, 35.7 mg; vitamin A, (–); vitamin B_1, 0.17 mg; vitamin B_2, 0.05 mg; niacin, 3.1 mg; vitamin C, (–).

BUCKWHEAT *(Fagopyrum esculentum)*

Buckwheat was probably first cultivated in central Asia, north of the Himalayas, and from there was taken to eastern Europe, China, and Japan. It is also known as Saracen corn and is thought to have been brought to Europe by the Crusaders. Buckwheat is not, in fact, botanically a grain: the plant is related to dock and rhubarb, and its fruit is a small, dark, three-sided nut that resembles a miniature beechnut. In Britain until recently it was cultivated mainly to feed pheasants and livestock, but in Russia and central Europe *kasha* (roasted buckwheat) is a popular staple food. There is a story told of a Russian Olympic team who arrived in Paris, couldn't find any buckwheat, and caught the next plane back to Moscow! Buckwheat "burgers" or croquettes are a popular alternative to the meat variety.

Buckwheat flour is difficult to extract from its sheathlike husks. As it is a heavy, dark flour it is often mixed with lighter rice or wheat flours, and is used for muffins or biscuits. In Japan the flour is used chiefly to make noodles called *soba*. These noodles are sometimes made from 100 percent buckwheat flour or more traditionally from 80 percent buckwheat and 20 percent whole wheat flours. They are a useful standby for your menus and can be added to soups (*see* Noodles). There has recently been an increase in the popularity of buckwheat pancakes. These are made in restaurants in France and other countries, but the batter is often prepackaged and can contain white sugar.

Buckwheat contains more protein than other grains as well as the amino acid lysine in which grains tend to be low. It is rich in iron and the B complex vitamins and is the best natural source of rutic acid, which helps arteries and circulatory ailments: For this reason homeopathic doctors prescribe it for high blood pressure and chilblains. It is also reportedly good for the lungs, kidneys, bladder, and water retention. It is definitely one of the more yang of the cereals, as it grows in very cold climates and the groats are small and compact. Evidently, insects do not attack it, and it fares poorly if chemicals are used on it. Although noodles can be eaten all year round, it is better to eat buckwheat groats more in the colder seasons as they generate body heat. Buckwheat is available in a roasted or unroasted form. To help the flavor re-roast for 5 minutes before cooking. The unroasted grains should be roasted in a dry skillet for 10 to 15 minutes. Stir to avoid burning.

Food Content of Buckwheat (per 100 g): calories, 335; protein, 11.7 g; fat, 2.4 g; carbohydrate, 72.5 g; fiber, 9.9 g; calcium, 33 mg; phosphorus, 282 mg; iron, 3.1 mg; sodium, 6.1 mg; potassium, 235 mg; vitamin A, (–); vitamin B_1, 0.6 mg; vitamin B_2, 0.15 mg; niacin, 4.4 mg; vitamin C, (–).

CORN OR MAIZE *(Zea mays)*

Corn is native to South America, where it has been used domestically for 10,000 years and has become the staple grain food and a source of flour or meal for the entire American continent. The name "corn" can cause confusion. To the English corn means wheat, to the Scots corn means oats, to the Americans it means corn on the cob. The reason for this is that when the early English settlers saw it they christened it Indian corn. The Indians worshiped the *Zea Mays* plant and called it "seed of seeds." Christopher Columbus introduced it to Europe where it became known by a variety of names: from "Turkish corn" in Germany and Holland to "Christian Corn" in Turkey! Today it is grown all over the world, from Argentina to Australia, from Asia to the plains of Italy. Corn needs hot sun and summer rainfall to flower and is more yin than the other cereals—bread from corn flour, cornmeal cakes, or popped corn do not make adequate staple food. The niacin content of corn is not released in the body. In Mexico and Peru they eat beans with their corn *tortillas*; in India they supplement their diet with lentils. During the Napoleonic wars in Europe, corn was the only food available and came to be associated with an epidemic of pellagra, a niacin-deficiency disease. This probably accounts for the fact that European farmers still regard corn mainly as animal food.

Corn makes a delicate corn syrup, corn oil, corn on the cob, and one particular variety is used to make popcorn. Bourbon is a product of fermented corn. Sweet corn (as it is called in England and Australia) or corn on the cob (in America) is grown as a vegetable but is much too sweet to be dried and ground into flour. The poorest corn, foodwise, is the most popular—popcorn.

The flour made from corn is often white and processed and although it is a good thickening agent it is not, nutritionally, of much value. Stoneground, whole grain, unsifted (unbolted) cornmeal is the type to buy. If it is whole grain it has not had the valuable germ removed. Cornmeal can be used as a supplementary grain to make desserts, breads, muffins, sauces, gravies, corn fritters, tempura batter, and the classic polenta. (*See* Recipe 57.)

Food Content of Corn (per 100 g): calories, 96; protein, 3.5 g; fat, 1.0 g; carbohydrate, 22.1 g; fiber, 0.7 g; calcium, 3 mg; phosphorus, 111 mg; iron, 0.7 mg; sodium, trace; potassium, 280 mg; choline, 112 mg; sulfur, 368 mg; vitamin A, 400 IU; vitamin B_1, 0.15 mg; vitamin B_2, 0.12 mg; niacin, 1.7 mg; vitamin C, 12 mg.

MILLET *(Panicum miliaccum)*

A native of Asia, millet once rivaled barley as the chief food of Europe and was more widely grown than wheat in the seventeenth and eighteenth centuries. In China it was a popular food before rice was introduced there, possibly around 2000 B.C. It is still a staple food in northern China, India, Korea, and Ethiopia. In Japan where it is also a traditional food it is called *awa* but is now used mainly for making millet *mochi* or to feed the parakeets! The most common millet in Britain is the bead-shaped, foxtail, Italian or yellow millet. Again it is the birds who benefit but in the West today millet is now coming under closer scrutiny as it is an essential food of the Hunzas, a remarkable tribe living in the Himalayan foothills, famed for their longevity and fitness.

Millet is a small, hard, and round grain; it is grown in cold climates and is the only yang, alkaline-forming grain. It is good for spleen or pancreas disorders and settles an acid stomach in no time! Millet lacks gluten, so that bread made from the flour does not rise very high but does have a good protein content. It contains more iron than any other cereal and is well balanced in amino acids.

Millet is a very versatile food and especially long lasting. It will keep, some reports say up to twenty years, and can be used in vegetable dishes, soups, stuffings, or cabbage rolls. It makes excellent croquettes (particularly with aduki beans), muffins, and pastries, or it can be eaten as a cereal. Its color is attractive and complements other foods well. As with most grains, millet should be washed and can be toasted before cooking.

To cook millet:

> 1 cup millet
> 4 to 5 cups water or vegetable stock
> Pinch of salt (per cup of millet)
> 1 teaspoon tamari or soy sauce

1. Place in pan, add water and salt, and bring to a boil.
2. Boil vigorously for 5 minutes. Lower heat, cover, and simmer for 30 to 40 minutes, or until water has disappeared. Do not stir or disturb grain.
3. Diced vegetables can be added—carrots and parsley for color, or onions.

Food Content of Millet (per 100 g): calories, 327; protein, 9.9 g; fat, 2.9 g; carbohydrate, 72.9 g; fiber, 3.2 g; calcium, 20 mg; phosphorus, 311 mg; sodium, (–); potassium, 430 mg; magnesium, 162 mg; iron, 6.8 mg; silicon, 160 mg; vitamin A, (–); vitamin B_1, 0.73 mg; vitamin B_2, 0.38 mg; niacin, 2.3 mg; vitamin C, (–).

OATS *(Avena sativa)*

Oats have been harvested since Neolithic times. They are native to Central Europe, and the wild oats common in Britain are thought to be the original ancestors of the modern cultivated variety. They are a staple food in Scotland, where they are thought to be good for the eyes. They are, in fact, rich in inositol, a B complex vitamin. Oats have one of the highest protein contents of all the grains. They are rich in calcium and iron. One brawny young Scot interviewed on TV declared that he ate oat porridge flavored with salt every day because it made him sexy! Oats do contain some zinc, which can help the male in that respect. Carl C. Pfeiffer gives the zinc content of oatmeal as 14 mg per 100 g. Oats have a high fat content, but they also contain soluble gums that bind cholesterol in the intestines, thus preventing its absorption. Oats have, in fact, been found effective in lowering the amount of cholesterol in the blood.

Rolled oats are generally used to make quick porridge. If they are marked "quick cooking" they have been precooked before they were rolled. *Oat flakes* may also be used for cereals, and as a basis for summer breakfast muesli, or for crumbles, cakes, and puddings. *Oat meals* are produced by various degrees of milling—fine, medium, and coarse. These can be used to make breads, creamy desserts, and "Bannocks" *(see Recipe 69)*, which are a tasty alternative to bread or toast. Cooked oats combine well with other cereals such as rice or millet to smooth a mixture for croquettes and to make soups creamy.

To make porridge it is quicker to use *steel cut oats,* although the most nutritious breakfast porridge is made with *whole oat groats.* They need thorough cooking (2 hours) but you can save time by soaking them 4 to 8 hours (the day before or overnight)—or try the following:

Ingredients

>1 cup whole oats
>5 to 6 cups water
>Pinch of ground kombu (or sea salt)
>1/2 cup oat milk

1. Wash the oats.

2. Place in a pot with water, sprinkle on kombu (or sea salt), and bring to a boil for 5 minutes.

3. Reduce heat to low, cover, and simmer for about 30 minutes, stirring from time to time to prevent sticking. Add more water if necessary. Turn off heat and leave covered overnight.

4. In the morning add milk and stir in. Simmer for 40 minutes or until smooth.

Pinhead oats are simpler: Bring 1 cup of oats in 4 cups water (with a pinch of kombu powder) to a boil, simmer for 30 minutes, then leave to stand covered overnight. Heat and simmer for 20 minutes before serving. Water or milk may need to be added. The whole oats can also be placed in boiling water and left, covered, in a very low 210°F oven overnight to be ready in the morning. Once made, porridge can be refrigerated and eaten cold or hot. If served cold, liquidize with stewed apple, raisin, and rice syrup. Serve with a little oat milk and sprinkle with grated almonds.

Food Content of Oats (per 100 g): calories, 313; protein, 13.0 g; fat, 5.4 g; carbohydrate, 66.1 g; fiber, 10.6 g; calcium, 55 mg; phosphorus, 320 mg; iron, 4.6 mg; sodium; potassium, (–); zinc, 14 mg; vitamin A, (–); vitamin B_1, 0.30 mg; vitamin B_2, 0.10 mg; niacin, 1.5 mg; vitamin C, (–).

RICE *(Oryza sativa)*

"Brown rice should be the staple of your diet. It is an excellent food, low in fat and rich in vitamins and minerals," says nutritionist Nan Bronfen. She is speaking from a scientific point of view. Rice, like wheat and many other cultivated grains, is native to the dry valleys of Central Asia. Interestingly enough early Chinese civilization didn't know rice at all—their staple grains were sorghum, wheat, and millet in the north, and yams in the swampy south. Aquatic rice is thought to have become established in India and to have reached China by 2000 B.C., spreading from there to Indonesia. Rice did not play a particularly important part in Japanese diet either until as late as the seventeenth century. Today more than half the world's population lives mainly on rice, and it is incredible that the rice eaten in many overpopulated areas should be commercially refined "white" rice, deprived of nourishing protein, calcium, iron, B vitamins, etc., lost when the valuable outer layers are removed. (*See* THE BODY—A LABORATORY, How Vital Are Vitamins?)

I remember craving a bowl of brown rice and vegetables during a stay in Hong Kong. I couldn't get it anywhere. I finally found a shop selling whole grain rice, took it back to the hotel and asked the waiter if they could cook some in the kitchen for me to eat in an hour's time. He looked astonished and explained that it would take much longer as he would have to polish each grain before it could be eaten! A Dr. Williams, who first extracted vitamin B_1 in an oil from rice bran, said, "Man commits a crime against nature when he eats the starch from the seed and throws away the mechanism necessary for the metabolism of that starch."

Whole grain or brown rice is referred to as "soul food" by Ohsawa who said it had the perfect balance of yin and yang. You are not expected to live on rice alone, but it will certainly be an important, central part of your diet. It is convenient for daily use, and it will help calm you when you are feeling edgy from dietary overindulgence or in times of stress or sickness. Learning to cook it well is, of course, one of the first lessons of macrobiotics. The principal varieties of rice available at most natural food stores are short-, medium, and long-grained rice. The harder, more compact short-grained rice is the more yang and is better suited for eating in cooler climates. Long-grained rice is better for warmer regions and hot weather. Cooked rice can be stored in a cool place or can be refrigerated, reheated, steamed, baked or fried, made into rice balls (croquettes), used in soups, salads, desserts, or breads, for sushi rolls, vegetable pies, casseroles, pilaf, paella, or stuffings.

Make sure your rice is whole grain and be careful when buying it—a large percentage of green grains means the rice is not ripe. Broken or chipped rice has been badly milled and cannot be stored for long as it will readily oxidize. Use organically grown rice if possible. It should say if it is organic on the package. If it doesn't, it isn't!

Whole grain rice takes longer to cook than do the commercial "white" varieties packaged for you in the supermarkets. The time it is cooking can be spent preparing the rest of the meal—the vegetables or sauce to go with it.

To cook brown rice:

>1 cup whole grain brown rice
>3 cups water
>Pinch of ground kombu (or sea salt)

1. Wash the rice. Place in a ceramic, stainless steel, cast iron or enamel pot—with a heavy lid preferably. Add water and kombu (or salt). It adds to the flavor and texture if you then soak for 2 or 3 hours. Bring to a boil.

2. Let the rice boil vigorously for 5 minutes, cover with the lid, lower the heat and simmer gently for 30 to 40 minutes, or until the water has disappeared. Do not stir or disturb the grain. If the heat is low it will not burn.

3. Turn off heat and, still covered, allow to stand for 10 minutes, or until ready to serve. Use a wooden ladle or spoon to serve.

Serve with a little tamari and sesame salt or a sauce made with sesame butter and miso.

To make the rice fluffier, the grains can first be dry roasted in an iron skillet or can be plunged directly into boiling water. In both cases the cooking time is slightly shorter.

A pressure cooker can also be used for brown rice. Use 2 cups of water to 1 cup of rice. Never fill cooker more than half full with grain.

Food Content of Brown Rice (per 100 g): calories, 360; carbohydrate, 77.4 g; fiber, 0.9 g; fat, 1.8 g; protein, 7.5. g; calcium, 32 mg; phosphorus, 220 mg; sodium, 9 mg; potassium, 216 mg; iron, 1.6 mg; sulfur, 10 mg; magnesium, 88 mg; selenium, 39 mg; copper, 0.2 mg; manganese, 1.6 mg; zinc, 1.8 mg; silicon, 40 mg; iodine, 0.002 mg; vitamin A, (–); vitamin B_1, 0.34 mg; vitamin B_2, 0.04 mg; vitamin B_6, 0.5 mg; niacin, 4.7 mg; vitamin C, (–).

RYE *(Secale cereale)*

Rye is probably of southwest Asian origin. In fertile soil it grows to seven to eight feet in height. To the Greeks it was a vigorous weed. The Romans began cultivating it. By the Middle Ages it was the staple grain throughout Europe, and the basic English loaf was made from roughly ground rye and barley. Germans still use it to make pumpernickel bread, and both Russians and Scandinavians prefer the flavor of dark whole rye bread. There are also "light" and "medium" rye flours available, which have been sifted and contain less bran. Commercial pumpernickel breads are often made with the "light," refined flour and are colored darker by the addition of caramel, molasses, instant coffee, or coffee substitutes. Always choose the least processed flour. In Scandinavia rye is used for crisp bread. Early settlers from Holland took rye seeds with them to America, where it is now used chiefly for animal food and is fermented to produce whisky. The Russians make beer from it.

Rye is similar in composition to wheat but is less glutenous; it is, though, more resistant to cold, disease, and pests. These are the only two grains that can be used by themselves to make bread. The protein in rye is less elastic, and the bread is heavier. But rye scores highly for taste. It is often mixed with wheat flour in bread recipes, and such bread is better if naturally leavened—up to 20 hours of slow rising. Rye can be made indigestible by leavening agents. There is a new high-protein grain called *triticale*, which is a cross between wheat and rye.

Rye is delicious mixed with rice. It is cooked the same way as rice and may be cracked with a rolling pin for faster cooking.

Food Content of Rye (per 100 g): calories, 334; carbohydrate, 73.4 g; fiber, 2.0 g; protein, 12.2 g; fat, 1.7 g; calcium, 38 mg; phosphorus, 376 mg; sodium, 1 mg; potassium, 467 mg; ; iron, 3.7 mg; sulfur, 28 mg; magnesium, 115 mg; silicon, 30 mg; iodine, 0.001 mg; vitamin A, (–); vitamin B_1, 0.43 mg; vitamin B_2, 0.22 mg; niacin, 1.6 mg; vitamin C, (–).

WHEAT *(Triticum aestivum/durum)*

Said to be native to Mesopotamia, wheat has been the "staff of life" and main food of temperate regions since recorded time. Egyptians, 4,000 years ago, isolated yeast and baked exotic, high-domed, coiled and plaited breads. Most of Cleopatra's "treacherous vessels" were used for carrying bread to Rome. Wheat seeds were taken to Britain and Gaul by the Romans, and a primitive variety of it, called *emmer* has been found in prehistoric village excavations in Britain. Columbus, in 1492, took wheat with him to the West Indies. Cortes, in 1519, took it to Mexico. The English distributed it to their colonies and shipped it to Australia, North America, and South Africa—and that versatile grass has flourished in all climates! There are many different varieties. In Canada the hard, red winter wheat, developed in drier areas and containing 11 to 15 percent protein, has the type of gluten best for making bread. The softer wheats from more humid areas, contain less protein (8 to 10 percent) and are usually used for cakes and pastries. Naturally, only flour from whole grains and preferably stoneground should be used. Macaroni, spaghetti, and other pasta products are made from the hard *durum* wheat semolina (semolina flour refers to the particles left after sifting out the fine white flour). *Couscous*, which is popular in North Africa, is made from wheat that is refined (but not bleached) and then cracked. It cooks very quickly. *Bulgur* is a form of whole wheat berries from which the outer, tough bran layer has been removed. The grain is then partially boiled, dried, and cracked; as it is partially precooked it can be eaten after boiling for 10 minutes or so. It is used extensively in the Middle East and features in salads. Bulgur and couscous are more yin and are better suited to hot climates.

White flour: Vicki Peterson in *The Natural Food Catalogue* tells of white flour, which was popular in the Middle Ages, when bakers treated it with chalk, alum, arsenic powder, and even ground-up bones from the graveyard! Today it is likely to be bleached with chlorine dioxide, which is also used to clean household drains!

Wheat germ: is not now generally recommended by nutritionists. It deteriorates rapidly, being high in fat, and is very likely to be rancid even if you purchase it freshly processed. Being a plant extract, it is yin and causes imbalance (*see* THE BODY—A LABORATORY, How Vital Are Vitamins?).

Whole wheat grain can be cooked. Soak first, overnight, then bring to a boil in 4 or 5 times the volume of water. Simmer for $1\frac{1}{2}$ hours, or until the grains have split open and are soft. They can then be made into croquettes mixed with rice or vegetables or added to soups. A traditional English dish called *frumenty* uses currants boiled with the cooked wheat.

Food Content of Hard Spring Wheat (per 100 g): calories, 330; carbohydrate, 69.1 g; fiber, 2.3 g; fat, 2.2 g; protein, 14 g; calcium, 36 mg; phosphorus, 383 mg; sodium, 3 mg; potassium, 370 mg; iron, 3.1 mg; magnesium, 160 mg; sulfur, 9 mg; silicon, 46 mg; iodine, 0.001 mg; bromine, 0.15 mg; vitamin A, (–); vitamin B_1, 0.57 mg; vitamin B_2, 0.12 mg; niacin, 4.3 mg; vitamin C, (–).

Hatcho Miso

(*See* Miso.)

Hijiki

(*See* Sea Vegetables.)

Kanten *(Agar-agar)*

This is a jellied dessert or aspic made from agar-agar, a healthy substitute for gelatin. Agar-agar sets firmer than gelatin and does not melt as readily. It needs to be used sparingly—1 to $1\frac{1}{2}$ teaspoons of flakes per 2 cups of liquid. Use fruit juice or flavor the water with corn syrup. Bring to a boil. Test a few drops on a cold plate before pouring the mixture into a wet bowl or jelly mold. If it sets too hard, kanten, unlike gelatin, can be reheated, have liquid added, and then allowed to reset.

Seasonal fruit can be used in the kantens—strawberries, cherries, blackberries, blueberries, peaches, pears, apples, raisins, etc. Melon should not need to be cooked—simply pour the hot juice and agar-agar mixture over it and allow it to set. Kanten can also be used to make a savory aspic by using vegetable stock or water and tamari with sliced vegetables, sea vegetables, fish, or aduki beans (*see also* Sea Vegetables).

Kasha or Buckwheat

(*See* Grains.)

Koji *(Aspergillus oryzae)*

This is a light green mold widely used for fermenting food products such as miso, shoyu, amazake, sake, and koji pickles. The role of koji is to trigger fermentation by providing nutrients needed by yeasts and bacteria. During its growth it produces enzymes that convert proteins, fats, and starches to simpler and more readily fermented substances. Koji is sensitive and reacts to small temperature and humidity changes. It thrives best at about 95°F, which is close to body temperature, and prefers a humidity of 80 percent. Koji can be purchased in some natural food stores.

Kombu

(*See* Sea Vegetables.)

Kome Miso

(*See* Miso.)

Kuzu

Kuzu is high-quality starch used as a thickener like arrowroot or as a very effective medicine. It is made from the root of the kuzu plant, which is native to the mountains of Japan and now grows wild in the southern United States, where it is called *kudzu*. It grows like a vine, wrapping itself around trees, often to a height of thirty feet. The tough roots grow deep into the ground, and the extraction of the starch from them is done by hand, which is a long and expensive process.

During early winter, when the sap and vitality of the plant is concentrated below, its roots are pulled from the soil. This work requires men, picks, shovels, winches, levers, and, at times, oxen, as some of the roots may have grown straight into mountains to a depth of fifteen or twenty feet. They can be several yards long, and as wide as a person. From them soft, white, chalklike kuzu is made; it contains more calories per gram than honey, but unlike honey, which is quick-burning sugar, kuzu is a long-sustaining source of energy and is easily digested. Although in appearance it resembles arrowroot, which is indigenous to tropical areas, it is a quite different product. It is usually packaged in small irregular lumps, which disperse quickly in cold water to make a milky liquid. When heated and stirred over low heat the liquid suddenly becomes clear. It makes an excellent thickener for Chinese-style vegetable sauces, it can be used in soups or in sweet jellies with kanten (*see* Kanten *and* Sea Vegetables). Kuzu helps digestion and since ancient times it has been popular in Japan as a treatment for colds and intestinal ailments. (For kuzu remedies *see* Umeboshi.)

Food Content of Kuzu (per 100 g): calories, 336; protein, 0.2 g; fat, 0.1 g; carbohydrate, 83.1 g; fiber, (–); calcium, 17 mg; phosphorus, 10 mg; iron, 2 mg; sodium, 2 mg; potassium, (–); vitamin A, (–); vitamin B_1, (–); vitamin B_2, (–); niacin, (–); vitamin C, (–).

Layering Method *(Nichime Style)*

This is a method of cooking vegetables, soups and stews in which the ingredients are placed in the pan with the more yin ones at the bottom and the more yang at the top. They are then allowed to cook, in a little water, undisturbed.

Legumes

Leguminous plants include peas and beans—seeds from a pod that opens lengthwise when ripe. Next to cereals they are the most vital source of human food. They contain many nutrients and more protein than any other vegetable product. They are a great protein booster when eaten with grains as they contain amino acids that cereals lack (*see* THE BODY—A LABORATORY, Protein Complements). They are useful in farming, as their roots harbor bacteria that convert nitrogen into nutrients that in turn enrich the soil. Members of the legume family include aduki beans, soybeans, black-eyed peas, pinto beans, mung beans, lentils, black turtle beans, red kidney beans, navy beans, lima beans, split peas, and garbanzos (or chickpeas). Peanuts are botanically classified as legumes, as are wisteria, laburnum, wild lupines, some poisonous weeds such as loco weed, and ornamentals such as the sweet pea.

Beans are also a good source of calcium, iron, and vitamins B_1 and niacin. Germinating bean sprouts, when the life force is activated within the seed by moisture and warmth, manufacture a rich source of nutrients needed for growth: amino acids and vitamins A, E, and B, including possibly vitamin B_{12}, which is so difficult to find in plant life. After a few hours of germination a seed develops vitamin C, which was completely lacking in its dry state. Certain beans can manufacture six times more vitamin C than can an equivalent amount of citrus fruit.

People sometimes complain that beans are difficult to digest, and there is a proverb in China that says, "A man who eats too many beans becomes a fool!" Too many can lead to irritability and unclear thinking, but if prepared and eaten properly, digestibility should really be no problem. Remember, the longer you soak and cook beans the softer and more digestible they are. The soaking time (changing the soaking water before cooking), the cooking time, and, as with all food, the chewing time are all important for proper digestion. Serve as a side dish rather than as the main food of the meal, or try adding them to grains, noodles, vegetables, or sea vegetables, even to fruit or raisins to make a dessert. Beans are interesting, too, when cooked together.

If they are properly stored in airtight containers in a cool place away from moisture and insects, beans can keep well for several years.

Preparing Legumes:

You are your own processor when it comes to preparing whole foods and, before cooking, beans should be spread on a cloth and sorted for any stones or bits and pieces, washed thoroughly, and soaked for an hour or more, sometimes overnight. Discard the soaking water. Another aid to their digestion is to place a couple of 2-inch strips of kombu or wakame sea vegetable in the pan. The beans should then be placed in fresh water (1 cup beans to 4 cups water), brought to a boil, covered, the heat reduced to low, and cooked for 40 minutes (depending on the type of bean—soybeans may need 4 hours or more). Then add 3 tablespoons of tamari or 1/4 teaspoon of sea salt or rock salt and cook, uncovered, for another 15 minutes, or until they are soft and most of the water has evaporated. If salt is added to the beans too early when cooking, the skins will harden.

When pressure cooking beans use only 3 cups of water to 1 cup of beans and halve the cooking time; remove the cover and add salt or tamari and cook, uncovered, until the liquid evaporates.

Legumes can be "shocked" during cooking. To avoid this, when adding cold water, pour the water slowly down the side of the pan.

Beans may also be baked. Boil them for 20 minutes first in 4 to 5 cups of water for each cup of beans. This will loosen their skins. Place a kombu strip in the baking dish, add water and beans, cover, and cook in a 350°F medium oven for 2 hours. You may need to add more water after a couple of hours. You can also add diced onions, carrots, or other root vegetables and can season with miso or tamari; alternately if you want to make a dessert, add raisins, apples, etc., during cooking.

ADUKI OR AZUKI BEANS *(Phaseolus angularis)*

The seeds of a "bushy" annual that is native to China and Korea were little known in the West until the advent of macrobiotics, but they are now being grown organically in Europe and America. In Japan the small, compact bean is called the "king of beans" and is said to be good for the liver and kidneys. Aduki is considered one of the more yang beans and can be used in soups, pies, pizzas, to make patés, or can be served with vegetables, sea vegetables, roasted pumpkin or sunflower seeds, etc. They make a nourishing and satisfying side dish, or they can be used with grains for croquettes.

Soak aduki for at least 1 hour, or even 2, before cooking. This will save cooking time. Cook as described above, with a strip of kombu, for $1^{1}/_{4}$ hours, then uncover, sprinkle with tamari and salt, increase heat, and cook another 20 minutes, or until most of the water has evaporated. Try diced carrot, pumpkin, or squash (marrow) added with the tamari for variety. In China and Japan aduki are used in desserts—try cooking them with 1 cup raisins per 1 cup of aduki. This makes a delicious kanten.

For kidney complaints boil 2 tablespoons of beans in 8 cups of water until soft ($1^{1}/_{2}$ hours). Add a dash of tamari, drain, and drink a little 3 times a day.

Food Content of Aduki Beans (dry) (per 100g): calories, 326; protein, 21.5g; fat, 1.6g; carbohydrate, 58.4g; fiber, 4.3g; calcium, 75mg; phosphorus, 350mg; iron, 4.8mg; sodium, 20mg; potassium, 1,500mg; vitamin A, 6 IU, vitamin B$_1$, 0.5mg; vitamin B$_2$, 0.1mg; niacin, 2.5mg; vitamin C, (–).

BLACK-EYED PEAS *(Vigna unguiculata)*

This bean has many names: cowpea, kaffir bean, Hindu cowpea, or yard-long bean (the asparagus cowpea, which has pods up to three feet in length). This legume has a distinctive black eye and originated in Africa, where it is still a staple food. Explorers took it to America and the West Indies in the seventeenth century, and it is very popular throughout the southern states of the United States. Today it is cultivated all over the tropical world. In Africa the dried seeds are roasted and ground into a coffee substitute, the young shoots eaten like spinach and the pod used as a green vegetable. Black-eyed peas become tender with cooking and absorb other flavors well.

Food Content of Black-eyed Peas (cooked) (per 100g): calories, 108; carbohydrate, 18 g; protein, 8.1 g; fat, 0.79 g; fiber, 4.3 g; calcium, 24 mg; phosphorus, 146 mg; sodium, 1.2 mg; potassium, 379 mg; iron, 2.1 mg; zinc, 1.8 mg; magnesium, 55 mg; vitamin A, 351 IU; vitamin B$_1$, 0.3 mg; vitamin B$_2$, 0.1 mg; niacin, 1.4 mg; vitamin C, 17 mg.

GARBANZOS/CHICKPEAS *(Cicer arietinum)*

Garbanzos is the Spanish name for chickpeas—also known as Egyptian peas, Bengal gram, *pois chiche*, and *ceci* (in Italy). These peas grow in curious hook-shaped pods and can be white, yellow, brown, red, or almost black. Their origin is rather uncertain. Chickpeas grew wild in Egypt at the time of the pharaohs. They are thought to have originated in western Asia and to have been introduced from there to Palestine and Mesopotamia and eastward to India. Explorers and merchants took them to Africa and South America. Today they are grown commercially as far abroad as Australia. They are a staple of the Middle East and are milled into flour, are roasted whole, or are ground after cooking and used to make *hummus* and *falafel* or deep-fried patties. Chickpeas also appear in many European and Oriental recipes.

Chickpeas need soaking for a long time—overnight is best. Use 2 cups of water per cup of peas. Pour away the soaking water and cook for 3 hours in 4 cups of fresh water. Add salt and simmer another hour. Be sure the water level is always above the beans otherwise they can be difficult to soften. It is a good idea to use a 2-inch strip of kombu when cooking them. As a variation, add diced onion with the salt for the last $\frac{1}{2}$ hour.

If pressure cooked, use 3 cups fresh water per cup of peas and cook for $1\frac{1}{2}$ hours.

Food Content of Garbanzos (dry) (per 100 g): calories, 360; carbohydrate, 61.0 g; fiber, 5 g; protein, 20.5 g; fat 4.8 g; fiber, 4.9 g; calcium, 150 mg; phosphorus, 331 mg; iron, 6.9 mg; sodium, 26 mg; potassium, 797 mg; sulfur, 110 mg; zinc, 2.7 mg; vitamin A, 50 IU; vitamin B_1, 0.31 mg; vitamin B_2, 0.15 mg; niacin, 2.0 mg; vitamin C, 5 mg; folic acid, 0.19 mg.

KIDNEY BEANS *(Phaseolus vulgaris)*

There are hundreds of different varieties of kidney-shaped beans: haricot beans, calico beans, navy beans, pinto beans, green and wax beans, snap beans, common beans, kidney beans or French beans, black turtle beans, *frijoles* or *spoca*. The American invention, baked beans in tomato sauce, sold in cans the world over, are haricot beans. "Boston beans" are a recipe made with pork by early American settlers from beans given to them by the friendly Indians who had cultivated kidney beans or French beans since prehistoric times. Columbus gave detailed descriptions of them growing in Cuba in 1492 and later, in Honduras, he saw the same plant with red or white seeds. These beans became a valuable source of nonperishable protein for sailors and explorers on such expeditions. The kidney bean was brought back to Europe in the sixteenth century and reached England through France in 1589 to be christened the French bean. These are the young pods and are prepared as a green vegetable. Snap beans have fibrous strings along the pod, which need to be removed before boiling. Navy beans are dry, mature seeds and have been developed to be resistant to disease. They are usually white in color. Black turtle beans are a shiny, black variety of the common kidney bean. They are a staple food throughout the Caribbean and Central and South America. Fried black beans and rice are the national breakfast dish of Costa Rica and are known as *galli pinto*. Cook with kombu to keep the skin from becoming too soft. All dried varieties of *Phaseolus vulgaris* are better cooked with kombu. Red kidney beans will have a creamier texture too if instead of adding tamari and salt for the last 20 minutes you place 1 or 2 teaspoons of miso (per cup of cooked beans) on top and cover with a lid. Mix only when cooking is completed.

Food Content of Red Kidney Beans (cooked) (per 100g): calories, 117; carbohydrate, 21.4 g; protein, 7.8 g; fiber, 1.5 g; fat, 0.5 mg; calcium, 37.8 mg; phosphorus, 140 mg; sodium, 3.2 mg; potassium, 340 mg; iron, 2.4 mg; copper, 0.34 mg; vitamin A, 5.4 IU; vitamin B_1, 0.1 mg; vitamin B_2, 0.05 mg; niacin, 0.7 mg; vitamin C, 3 mg; folic acid, 0.03 mg.

LENTILS *(Lens esculenta)*

The biblical "mess of pottage" that Jacob gave Esau was made of lentils, one of the earliest cultivated crops in the East. It would seem that a traveling Seventh Day Adventist from Germany introduced them to America when he gave some to an obviously enterprising farmer who proceeded to cultivate them.

There are many different varieties of lentils, usually identified by their color—green, red, orange, yellow, brown, or black. They play an important part in Indian cooking in various types of *dal*. Lentils are richer in protein than any of the other legumes except soybeans. The pink and red varieties from

India contain more protein than do the other types. In third world countries their calorific value has earned them the name of "poor man's meat."

Lentils do not need much soaking. They cook comparatively quickly—in 30 minutes. Add 1/4 teaspoon of sea salt and cook an additional 10 minutes, or until most of the water has evaporated.

Food Content of Lentils (cooked) (per 100 g): calories, 106; protein, 27.8 g; fat, trace; carbohydrate, 19.3 g; fiber, 1.2 g; calcium, 25 mg; phosphorus, 119 mg; iron, 2.1 mg; sodium, 30 mg; potassium, 249 mg; copper, 0.27 mg; zinc, 1.0 mg; vitamin A, 20 IU; vitamin B_1, 0.07 mg; vitamin B_2, 0.06 mg; niacin, 0.6 mg; vitamin C, (–).

LIMA BEANS *(Phaseolus lunatus)*

There are several varieties of lima bean and they come in two sizes: the larger is the butter bean and the smaller is called the sieva bean. Other names for it are curry bean or pole bean. Apparently, lima beans were discovered in pre-Inca tombs in Peru dated 5000 B.C. and were common in America when Columbus arrived there. The Spanish conquistadores took them to the Philippines, and by the seventeenth century the lima bean was growing in hot areas all over the world. It is still, today, the main legume crop of tropical Africa and is called Madagascar bean there. It has never survived colder regions and has to be imported into the United Kingdom and Europe, where "butter beans" have long been popular canned, dried, or frozen. The white beans are usually preferred, probably because raw lima seeds contain a poisonous element, *organogenetic glycoside*, and the white bean is considered less toxic than the darker types. Prolonged soaking and boiling removes this toxin. Being a tropical bean it is considered, with soy beans, the most yin of the legume family. It is a good idea to toast them in a dry skillet and soak them overnight before cooking with a yang vegetable such as burdock root or lotus root. They shouldn't be eaten too often and must be chewed well.

Food Content of Lima Beans (cooked) (per 100 g): calories, 138; carbohydrate, 25.6 g; protein, 8.20 g; fiber, 1.6 g; fat 0.6 g; calcium, 29 mg; phosphorus, 154 mg; sodium, 2.7 mg; potassium, 612 mg; iron, 3.1 mg; zinc, 0.89 mg; copper, 0.57 mg; vitamin A, 30 IU; vitamin B_1, 0.13 mg; vitamin B_2, 0.05 mg; niacin, 0.68 mg; vitamin B_6, 0.18 mg; vitamin C, 1 mg; folic acid, 0.04 mg.

MUNG BEANS *(Phaseolus mungo* or *vigna mungo)*

In India, where this bean was cultivated before recorded history, it is known as *moong dal* and is used to make flour. This bean is popular throughout Asia today. In the East it is made into porridge with a little glutinous rice. Indonesians use it against protein deficiency and, in Malaya, large quantities of mung bean gruel are consumed after the Ramadan month of fasting. In China it is the small green type that is commonly sprouted and used to make noodles.

As they can contain up to 37 percent protein and are considered a rich source of vitamin B_2 and vitamin C, mung bean sprouts are useful—and delicious—served cold in salads or cooked with vegetable dishes. In India the rare *black gram bean* is important among the high castes, and the golden seed is gaining popularity in America and Europe.

Food Content of Mung Bean Sprouts (raw) (per 100 g): calories, 35.2; protein, 3.8 g; fat 0.2 g; carbohydrate, 6.6 g; fiber, 0.67 g; calcium, 19 mg; phosphorus, 64 mg; iron, 1.3 mg; sodium, 5 mg; potassium, 223 mg;

zinc, 0.86 mg; vitamin A, 19 IU; vitamin B$_1$, 0.13 mg; vitamin B$_2$, 0.13 mg; niacin, 0.76 mg; vitamin C, 19 mg; folic acid, 0.008 mg.

PEAS *(Pisum sativum)*

The common garden pea, *petit pois*, snow pea, or marrow fat pea, is marketed according to its size and sugar and starch content. Split peas are the dried peas without their skins. This annual climber prefers northern climates but can also be grown in more tropical areas. The history of the pea is, in fact, one of the longest and most illustrious of the legumes. Some historians even believe it originated in the Garden of Eden—that is, between the Euphrates and Tigris Rivers. Remains of it have been found in the ruins of Troy, in predynastic Egyptian tombs, and at the site of a Neolithic lake village in Switzerland dated 4500 B.C. The Greeks prized it, the Romans cultivated it, it spread to Abyssinia and Africa, reaching Asia by A.D. 400. From there is was taken east to India and west to Europe where, by the Middle Ages, it was one of the most important legumes. In the seventeenth century, at the court of Louis XIV, aristocrats were consuming large platefuls of fresh, young green peas after visiting the theater, according to Madame de Maintenon's diary! The French fashion caught on in England and peas are popular as a green vegetable to this day. Unfortunately they are more often canned or frozen and are likely to contain green coloring and sugar. This is because of "popular demand" say the manufacturers! Split peas have held their own and cook more quickly than other legumes. Soak them overnight. *Petit pois* are the very young, small peas that have a lower starch content. They are used in freezing and canning.

Food Content of Split Peas (cooked) (per 100 g): calories,115; protein, 8 g; fat, 0.15 g; carbohydrate, 20.8 g; fiber, 0.4g; calcium, 11 mg; phosphorus, 89 mg; iron, 1.7 mg; sodium, 13 mg; potassium, 296 mg; copper, 0.25 mg; vitamin A, 40 IU; vitamin B$_1$, 0.15 mg; vitamin B$_2$, 0.09 mg; niacin, 0.9 mg; vitamin C, (–).

Food Content of Green Peas (cooked) (per 100 g): calories, 71.3; protein, 5.4 g; fat, 0.4 g; carbohydrate, 12.1 g; fiber, 2 g; calcium, 23 mg; phosphorus, 98.8 mg; iron, 1.8 mg; sodium, 1.3 mg; potassium, 136.3 mg; copper, 0.15 mg; zinc, 0.75 mg; vitamin A, 538 IU; vitamin B$_1$, 0.28 mg; vitamin B$_2$, 0.11 mg; vitamin B$_6$, 0.15 mg; niacin, 2.3 mg; pantothenic acid, 0.34 mg; vitamin C, 20 mg.

SOYBEANS *(Clycine max)*

The seeds of the soybean are small and oval in shape and vary in color from yellow to gray and brown to black. The bean, also known as *haba soya* or *preta*, is native to China and for thousands of years has been called "the meat of the earth" in the Far East. Modern analysis has proved the title an apt one: the soybean is one of the few sources of so-called high-quality plant protein. It is an outstanding protein booster and can increase usable protein substantially when eaten with grains, which have a shortage of lysine (*see* THE BODY—A LABORATORY, Protein Complements). Soybeans were first recorded in 2800 B.C. by the Emperor Shen Nung, who described them as one of the most important crops in his country. Use of the bean spread to Japan and Korea. It was taken to Europe in 1712 and samples were grown in the hothouses of Kew Gardens in England, but not until the twentieth century did the bean begin to be produced commercially in the West. By 1969 the American government had subsidized over 41 million acres for soybean cultivation. America now leads, with China, in commercial soybean production, which has become big business not only as food but for industrial use as well. Paint manufacture, the plywood industry, brewing, pharmaceutical and cosmetic products all utilize the natural emulsifying and binding properties of soybean extracts, while their natural preservative qualities are valuable in prolonging the shelf life of various foodstuffs. Soybeans are used to produce flour, oil, textured vegetable and meat-substitute protein as well as the valuable traditional fermented foods such as miso, tofu, tempeh, and tamari. (see INGREDIENTS). Soy milk is often made with added sugar, so check your labels. In 1997 there were suggestions of genetic manipulation to make the soybean more insect resistant; check too, that your product is made from organic beans. Soy yogurt, whipped cream, and even cheese are are also now available on various world markets.

The soybean is considered the most yin of the pulses and is not recommended for frequent use. Nutritionist Nan Bronfen warns that it is higher in fat than most legumes and has a rich lecithin level (see THE BODY— A LABORATORY, Facts About Fats). Soybean sprouts should never be eaten uncooked (steam or stir-fry for 6 or 8 minutes) because the raw bean contains a substance known as trypsin inhibitor, which seems to interfere with protein digestion and the assimilation of the amino acid methionine in the body. This also applies to sprouted peas, chickpeas, beans, fenugreek, alfalfa, and lentils. Grain sprouts can be eaten raw.

Before cooking soybeans it is a good idea to roast them in a skillet and soak them for 24 hours (3 cups water per cup of beans), bring to a boil in fresh water with kombu and simmer for 2 to 4 hours. Add flavorings during the last hour. If pressure cooking soybeans, add a teaspoon of vegetable oil (corn, soy, sesame, or sunflower) to keep the skin from clogging the gauge! Black soy or Japanese beans can be soaked with 1/2 teaspoon of salt added to the water to prevent the skin from coming off the beans. Change the water, bring to a boil, and simmer. Skim off any gray foam that floats to the top. When foam no longer appears, cover the pot and cook for 2 1/2 to 3 hours. Add a little tamari and shake the pot.

Food Content of Cooked Soy Beans (per 100 g): calories, 130; protein, 11.0 g; fat 5.7 g; carbohydrate, 10.7 g; fiber, 1.7 g; calcium, 72.8 mg; phosphorus, 179 mg; iron, 2.7 mg; sulfur, 265 mg; sodium, 2.2 mg; potassium, 540 mg; vitamin A, 27.8 IU; vitamin B_1, 0.21 mg; vitamin B_2, 0.1 mg; niacin, 0.6 mg; vitamin C, (–). (The vitamin C content of soybean sprouts is 13.3 mg.)

Lotus Root (Nelumbium muciferum)

The lotus is a sacred plant in India and China and is used extensively for cooking in the Far East. The lotus root is actually a tuber that grows horizontally in the mud bottoms of ponds and mysteriously retains pockets of air. The root is brown outside, the hollow-chambered inside is off-white. The perforated pattern is decorative for many dishes. Lotus is one of the more yang roots and is especially good for respiratory problems. It is traditionally used for colds, sinus and lung congestion, etc. Lotus root tea is made by grating the fresh root and squeezing out the juice, adding an equal quantity of water, a pinch of grated ginger, and a pinch of sea salt. Bring these ingredients to a boil and simmer for 2 to 3 minutes. Powdered lotus tea from a natural food store may be used instead. Dried roots are available but need soaking in water first.

Food Content of Fresh Lotus (per 100 g): calories, 62; protein, 2.4 g; fat, 0.1 g; carbohydrate, 14.3 g; fiber, 0.9 g; calcium, 20 mg; phosphorus, iron, 0.5 mg; sodium, 30 mg; potassium; vitamin B_1, 0.05 mg; vitamin B_2, 0.03 mg; niacin, 0.5 mg; vitamin C, 20 mg.

Maple Syrup

Maple syrup is made from the sap of maple trees in the northern United States and Canada. It takes about 200 quarts (200 liters) of sap to make 1 gallon of syrup. It is a natural sweetener, but use it in moderation. It is useful when changing from sugars to something less sweet.

Food Content of Maple Syrup (per 100 g): calories, 250; protein, (–); fat, (–); carbohydrate, 6 g; calcium, 165 mg; phosphorus, 15 mg; iron, 1 mg; sodium, 15 mg; potassium, 130 mg; copper, 0.45 mg; vitamin A, (–); vitamin B_1, (–); vitamin B_2, (–); niacin, (–); vitamin C, (–).

Mirin

Mirin is a natural sweetening agent used in cooking and made from sweet rice, rice koji (a cultivating rice mold), and spring water. It is used in broths, dips, salad dressing, and marinades for tofu or fish. It is sometimes served hot with Mu tea.

Miso

The story of a whole culture is contained in the name miso. There are early references in Chinese literature to a type of miso that could contain a mixture of meat or fish and sometimes sweet, wild fruit. It was eaten in the Orient long before the Christian era. The first reference to soybeans used as a protein source was in A.D. 500, by which time Buddhism was encouraging a meatless diet and the monks developed a process of salt pickling and fermentation that showed a remarkable understanding of microbiology. Some scholars maintain that the origins of miso are in the heartland of northern Japan, where ancient homemade miso traditions are still very much in practice. The miso is still allowed to age in cedar vats without haste for eighteen months to three years by the same process of enzymatic fermentation that has been used for centuries. Miso is made from cooked soybeans or cooked rice, barley, wheat, buckwheat, whole rice, or white rice, which has koji added, and sea salt to spur the growth of the fungus that produces enzymes that digest starches and proteins during the lengthy fermentation process. The difference between types of miso is due, in part, to the different kojis used to make them. After World War II, stainless steel, fast fermentation, and mass production drastically changed the quality—and flavor—of miso. However, there were men in Japan who fortunately, like the many small vintners in France, held on to the natural and traditional production methods. These men waited patiently for the fad for fast food to pass. As people have begun to object to the taste of chemicals and synthetics, traditional miso is again becoming popular.

Miso paste is an essential ingredient in macrobiotic cooking, and you will soon grow to rely on it. It is high in protein, including all the essential amino acids and calcium; it is free of toxins and the enzymes and bacteria in it help proper digestion. Miso is also a source of vitamin B_{12}, which is an important supplement for vegetarians (*see also* Soybeans).

HATCHO MISO

This is a soybean miso made from soybean koji. Known as the food of the samurai warriors, it is made according to a recipe more than 400 years old. The cooked soybeans are inoculated with koji (*Aspergillus oryzae*). Hatcho is very dry miso and is made in enormous cedarwood kegs with less water and less salt than red or barley misos. It ferments slowly and needs over three years to mature under heavy pressure. Hatcho is the thickest in texture of the misos and has a rich, almost chocolate-like taste that goes well with the darker, heavier root and winter vegetables. It is an excellent base for miso soups, or it can be mixed with other kinds of miso to subtly change flavors.

Food Content of Hatcho Miso (per 100 g): calories, 180; protein, 16.8 g; fat, 6.9 g; carbohydrate, 15.8 g; fiber, 2.2 g; calcium, 140 mg; phosphorus, 240 mg; iron, 6.5 mg; sodium, 3,800 mg; potassium, (–); vitamin B_1, 0.04 mg; vitamin B_2, 0.12 mg; niacin, 1.2 mg; vitamin B_{12}, 0.17 mg; vitamin C, (–).

MUGI MISO

This means barley miso and is made with barley koji. It is called the "country-style" miso and is popular because it is suitable for both summer and winter cooking. The pleasing aromas of mugi may also account for its popularity. The barley koji is mixed with the soybeans in kegs to ferment. Barley, which contains both proteins and starches, produces the enzymes to reduce protein to amino acids and produces other enzymes to convert starches to sugars, which are further fermented to produce alcohols and ethers—which is why mugi smells so good!

KOME MISO

Kome means, in most cases, "white rice." But there are several different kinds of kome miso, and they are the most generally used in Japan. Rice koji works primarily to convert starches to sugars, and the fermentation is more active and rapid. It is the same kind of koji as that used to make amazake, sake, and rice vinegar. Kome is the sweetest of the misos. There are many different varieties: *Shiro* (white) miso is the sweetest and can be made in one or two weeks. It spoils quickly if not refrigerated but is a beautiful summer miso and can be used for salad dressings, sauces, and spreads. There are other types of rice misos, all various shades of red *(aka* miso), orange, and brown and each with a different flavor. Kome misos go well with lighter vegetables and greens in the spring and summer.

GENMAI MISO

This is a kome or rice miso but a more modern type, which has been produced since brown rice came into demand. *Genmai* means "brown rice." Traditionally, white rice is used to make nearly all rice misos because the outer bran of brown rice is resistant to any kind of spoilage or molds—including koji! The result of recent experimentation is the richly flavored genmai miso.

NATTO MISO

This is made from soybeans and ginger.

SOBA MISO

This is made from buckwheat.

Miso soup is a good energy booster when there is work to be done and makes a light and nourishing meal at any time of the day but, before being added to soups, casseroles, stews, etc., miso needs to be ground into a purée. Your suribachi is perfect for this. Add a little soup stock or hot water (1/2 cup to a tablespoon of miso) and stir it well before adding it to the soup.

Miso should not generally be boiled and the pot should be taken off the heat when the miso is added or, preferably, the miso puree mixed in each bowl, then stirred in the soup when serving. I find that if the miso has boiled the soup can taste sour when reheated later. Manufacturers certainly recommend that it is not boiled for long periods except in special kinds of cooking.

Try to resist the temptation to use too much miso. It is delicious but is also a very yangizing ingredient.

Mochi

Mochi is rice cake generally made from cooked, pounded sweet rice, which is more glutinous than regular brown rice. In Japan sweet rice is traditionally used to make the alcoholic drink sake. It is also used in making mochi.

Mochi can also be made from a sweet millet or millet and sweet rice mixture, or by adding dry-roasted black soybeans during the final stages of pounding. Fresh mugwort may also be pounded into the rice. Mochi can be purchased ready-made in a variety of flavors.

Pan-fry squares of Mochi over low heat or bake in the oven until it puffs up. Serve with a seasoning of tamari and ginger juice. Delicious served in miso soup.

Food Content of Rice Mochi (cooked) (per 100 g): calories, 336; protein, 7.6 g; fat, 2.3 g; carbohydrate, 73.2 g; fiber, 1.2 g; calcium, 10 mg; phosphorus, 290 mg; iron, 1.1 mg; sodium, 3 mg; potassium, (–); vitamin B_1, 0.36 mg; vitamin B_2, 0.10 mg; niacin, 4.5.

Natto

Natto is another soybean-ferment product high in protein, calcium, and iron, which aids the digestion of food in the intestines. Wendy Esko, in *Introducing Macrobiotic Cooking,* says that she notices that eating natto also makes the skin feel smooth and young. "A person who has eaten much dairy food, " she observes, "is more likely to dislike natto than someone who has been macrobiotic for several years and has discharged much of his past dairy food intake."

Natto can be served on buckwheat noodles or with tamari over a bowl of rice. It is sold in small frozen packets.

Food Content of Natto (per 100 g): calories, 167; protein, 16.9 g; fat, 7.4 g; carbohydrate, 11.5 g; fiber, 3.2 g; calcium, 103 mg; phosphorus, 182 mg; iron, 3.7 mg; sodium, (–); potassium, 249 mg; vitamin B_1, 0.07 mg; vitamin B_2, 0.5 mg; niacin, 1.1 mg.

Natto Miso

This is not actually a miso but is a condiment made by briefly fermenting soybeans, grains, ginger, and kombu.

Nigari

Nigari is hard, crystallized salt made from dampened sea salt. It is used in making tofu.

Nori

(*See* Sea Vegetables.)

Noodles

It is said that Marco Polo took the idea of kneading dough, stretching it, rolling it, and cutting it into long strands from China to Italy and started the Italian pasta tradition. Before that though, traveling monks in the ninth and tenth centuries brought the idea from China to Japan, and Japanese noodles emerged to stay. They are generally made using buckwheat, whole wheat, or rice flours, which certainly are healthier than the white flour spaghetti products in our Western supermarkets.

Noodles are quickly and easily prepared and just what you need for unexpected guests; they are a favorite, all-year-round food that can be used for breakfast, lunch, dinner, or as a snack. They can be eaten hot, once cooked, or can be served cold. They can be fried with vegetables, tempuraed, served simply with tamari and chopped scallions, or in a broth. There are several varieties of noodles.

SOBA NOODLES

Soba means "buckwheat." It also means "close by." In Japan it is a custom to present soba noodles to new neighbors as a gift of welcome and a bowl of soba is traditionally eaten at the New Year. Soba is so popular that the demand for it exceeds its domestic production, and a great deal of the flour is imported from Canada and Brazil. As buckwheat contains almost no gluten and does not lend itself to the making of pasta, soba noodles are normally made from 80 percent buckwheat flour with 20 percent whole wheat flour, but there is also a 100 percent buckwheat noodle. Other soba noodles are *ftoh* soba, a short, thin soba noodle; *jenenjo* soba, which contains *jenenjo* flour made from a mountain potato of that name; *cha* soba, which contains tea leaves; and *youmugi* soba, which is made by using mugwort.

Cooking soba properly requires a good-sized pot so that the noodles won't stick together. They already contain salt, so very little needs to be added.

1. Bring water to a boil and add noodles. Bring to a boil again. Stir to keep them from sticking together. After a minute a head of foam will begin to rise.
2. Add a small amount of water to stop the boiling. Bring to a boil again.
3. Repeat this 3 times. Reduce heat and allow the noodles to simmer for about 7 minutes. Stir well.
4. Strain them under running cold water to prevent sticking. Reheat by using a little soy, olive, or sesame oil in the bottom of the pan.

An alternative method is to place soba in boiling water, bring to a boil again, lower heat, and simmer for 10 to 15 minutes. Strain in running, cold water. When cooked, the noodle should be the same color throughout when broken. Or try the old Italian spaghetti test of throwing a piece against a smooth wall—if it sticks it's cooked! The water used for cooking soba can be seasoned and served as a drink *(sobaya),* either hot or cold.

Food Content of Soba (cooked) (per 100 g): calories, 360; protein, 10.8 g; fat, 1.8 g; carbohydrate, 73 g; fiber, 0.4 g; calcium, 30 mg; phosphorus, 210 mg; iron, 5.0 mg; sodium, 700 mg; potassium, (–); vitamin B_1, 0.2 mg; vitamin B_2, 0.88 mg; niacin, 1.2 mg, vitamin C, (–).

UDON NOODLES

Udon is plain wheat pasta and comes from the wheat district, the island of Shikoku. It is traditionally made from refined, "sifted" flour but is obtainable now from 80 percent whole wheat and 20 percent "sifted" flour There is also a 100 percent whole wheat udon noodle and a rice udon noodle.

Udon, like soba, is best cooked in plenty of water and in the same way. It takes a little longer, say 5 more minutes, to cook. It need not be washed but can be scooped straight from the pot. If cooked too long, however, it may need to be rinsed in cold water.

The noodle water from cooking udon can be used for noodle broth, stews, etc.

SOMEN NOODLES

These are a light, very thin noodle. They are dried outside in the icy cold of winter and are usually served cold in the summer.

Food Content of Somen (per 100 g): calories, 341; protein, 8.4 g; fat, 1.3 g; carbohydrate, 71.8 g; fiber, 0.3 g; calcium, 24 mg; phosphorus, 110 mg; iron, 1.8 mg; sodium, 1,200 mg; potassium, (–); vitamin B_1, 0.12 mg; vitamin B_2, 0.04 mg; niacin, 1.0 mg.

RAMEN NOODLES

These are Chinese-style noodles that have become popular. There is an instant variety, precooked in hot oil and sometimes chicken fat, which disqualifies them as natural food! But there is also a variety of crinkly, whole grain Ramen made by a steam and bake method that is oil free. These make delicious soups.

SAIFUN NOODLES

These are a clear "cellophane" noodle made from mung beans.

There are of course other whole grain noodles available that will add variety to your menus: spaghetti, shells, rigatoni, spirals, flat noodles, lasagna, and so forth. They are sometimes available made of whole wheat flour and are generally made without salt.

Probably the most important ingredient for noodle dishes is the broth in which they are served (*see* Dashi). There are several sauces that can be made (*see* RECIPES—Sauces).

Nuts

Botanically, nuts are the single seeds or edible kernels of plants and have a hard or brittle shell. The Greeks used them, the Romans cultivated them and sugared them. Medieval Europeans learned from the Arabs to use them for sweetmeats, and the Moors taught the Spanish, who in turn took their recipes to the Americas after the conquest where the Aztecs were already using pumpkin seeds, peanuts, and probably pecans to thicken sauces. Nuts contain rich quantities of minerals and vitamins, they are high in protein but have a large stock of oil to be used as energy needed by the new plant life that will spring from them.

Their shells protect them from heat, air, light, and moisture almost indefinitely. Once shelled, on the other hand, the oil in them quickly oxidizes and becomes rancid. They should be stored, tightly covered, in a cool, dark, dry place. It is advisable to buy them unshelled as packaged, commercial nuts can be treated with preservatives, dyes, and inhibitors and are often fried in saturated or rancid fats. Try to find a reputable organic source. Most nutritionists advise against eating too many—no more than half a dozen a day. Toasting the kernels is a good idea. Nuts are more yin, toasting is yang and

63

certainly brings out their flavor. Use the skillet (no oil) for 5 to 10 minutes, or place them in a medium oven for 15 minutes.

Use nuts sparingly as a condiment, for decoration, or to flavor kantens, cakes, etc.

ALMONDS (Prunus dulcis)

Almonds are the seeds of a tree of the peach family, native to the eastern Mediterranean. In early spring groves of the pink and white blossoms adorn the landscapes of the regions in which it grows. The ladies of Rome used almond oil as a skin moisturizer and today it is still an ingredient in beauty creams. There are two varieties: sweet and bitter. Sweet almonds are used whole or ground or are pounded into a milky paste. They can be sliced or "slivered" and added as a flavoring for soups or fish dishes. Almonds also combine well with chicken and rice or they can be baked and salted with tamari. Bitter almonds are broader in shape and their powerful flavor, similar to peach or plum kernels, is due to an enzyme reaction that produces prussic acid. This poison fortunately evaporates when heated, but *raw* bitter almonds should be avoided.

Food Content of Almonds (cooked) (per 100 g): calories, 598; protein, 18.6 g; fat, 52.2 g; carbohydrate, 19.5 g; fiber, 2.6 g; calcium, 234 mg; phosphorus, 504 mg; iron, 4.3 mg; sodium, 4 mg; potassium, 773 mg; magnesium, 271 mg; copper, 0.83 mg; manganese, 1.9 mg; vitamin B_1, 0.2 mg; vitamin B_2, 0.92 mg; niacin, 3.5 mg; vitamin B_6, 0.1 mg; biotin, 17.6 mg; folic acid, 0.1 mg; pantothenic acid, 0.47 mg; vitamin C, trace; vitamin E, 15.0 mg.

BRAZIL NUTS (Bertholettia excelsa)

These are the seeds of a tall forest tree in South America, and collecting them can be a risky business. In high winds those who gather them need to wear protective headgear as each shell, the size of a coconut, can weigh up to four pounds. Inside this shell the Brazil nuts are packed away neatly like chocolates in a box! Surprisingly few of the nuts are, in fact, consumed in Brazil where, to quote "Charley's Aunt," "the nuts come from!" Half the crop goes to the United States, where their popularity continues to increase, and they have been taken to Europe since 1633. They can be roasted, used in cakes, or grated on vegetables or kantens.

Food Content of Brazil Nuts (per 100 g): calories, 654; protein, 14.3 g; fat, 66.9 mg; carbohydrate, 10.9 g; fiber, 3.1 g; calcium, 186 mg; phosphorus, 693 mg; iron, 3.4 mg; sodium, 1 mg; potassium, 715 mg; magnesium, 251 mg; copper, 1.5 mg; manganese, 2.8 mg; zinc, 5.1 mg; selenium, 102 mg; vitamin B_1, 0.96 mg; vitamin B_2, 0.12 mg; niacin, 1.6 mg; folic acid, 0.004 mg; pantothenic acid, 0.23 mg; vitamin C, 10 mg; vitamin E, 6.5 mg.

CASHEW NUTS (Anacardium occidentali)

The South American Indians called the fruit of this tree native to Brazil *acaju*, which Portuguese colonists heard as *caju*. The Portuguese took the cashew to their Indian colonies in the sixteenth century, and India is now one of the biggest exporters of the nut. The fruit of the cashew is fleshy, tart, reddish, and pear shaped and is called an apple. The nut grows as a hard protuberance under this fruit, and although the kernel is edible, there is a toxic oil in the outer layer that produces blisters on contact with the skin. This layer must be removed and the nut roasted before it is eaten. In fact, many

Brazilians simply detach the cashew nut and eat the fruit! Cashew nuts are mainly used salted (and roasted), in baking, or to make cashew butter or cream. They are also tasty as a condiment on green vegetables or as a decoration for meat dishes.

Food Content of Cashew Nuts (roasted) (per 100 g): calories, 561; protein, 17.2 g; fat, 45.7 mg; carbohydrate, 29.3 g; fiber, 1.4 g; calcium, 38 mg; phosphorus, 373 mg; iron, 3.8 mg; sodium, 15 mg; potassium, 464 mg; magnesium, 267 mg; zinc, 4.35 mg; vitamin B_1, 0.43 mg; vitamin B_2, 0.25 mg; niacin, 1.8 mg; folic acid, 0.06 mg; pantothenic acid, 1.3 mg.

CHESTNUTS *(Castanea sativa)*

Sweet chestnuts should not be confused with horse chestnuts *(Aesculus hippocastanum)*, which are more suitable as squirrel food. *Castanea sativa* is native to the Mediterranean and belongs to the same family as the oak and beech. Roman legions carried it to colder, northern regions beyond the Alps, where it grows quite happily, but the fruit will not ripen. Spain being the traditional source of the sweet chestnut in Britain, it is known there as *Spanish chestnut*. In France, where probably the highest quality of nut is produced, it is called *marron*, and *marron glacé* is a famous sweet. In Italy, however, it is a staple food and is ground into a flour, *farina dolce*, which is used to make bread and gruel.

The chestnut does not keep well at room temperature. Treat it more like a vegetable. It contains more carbohydrate and much less oil than do most nuts. It can be served roasted, boiled, steamed, pureed, or used in pies or stuffings; the flour makes delicious bread. To peel sweet chestnuts, place them in boiling water, turn off the heat, and let stand for 5 minutes. Remove and allow to cool. Then peel with a sharp knife. To roast them, remember to slit the outer casing on the flat side and place on a baking tray, flat side up, in a medium oven (or in front of a wood fire!) for 20 minutes or so. Test for tenderness by inserting a knife through the slit.

Food Content of Chestnuts (per 100 g): calories,19; protein, 2.9 g; fat, 66.9 mg; carbohydrate, 42.1 g; fiber, 1.1 g; calcium, 27 mg; phosphorus, 88 mg; iron, 1.7 mg; sodium, 6 mg; potassium, 454 mg; magnesium, 53.61 mg; copper, 3.6 mg; vitamin B_1, 0.22 mg; vitamin B_2, 0.22 mg; niacin, 0.6 mg; vitamin A, 89 IU; vitamin B_6, 0.33 mg; biotin, 1.3 mg; pantothenic acid, 0.47 mg; vitamin C, 6 mg; vitamin E, 0.5 mg.

HAZELNUTS *(Corylus avellana)* and FILBERTS *(Corylus maxima)*

The name "hazelnut" is from the Anglo Saxon word *haesil*, which means headdress; this describes precisely how this nut fits into its cupule or covering. Filberts, on the other hand, which are longer and more robust, are named after a French abbot, St. Philbert, whose feast day in August coincides with their time of ripening. Hazelnuts are more common in Europe, and filberts more usual in the United States. Both are high in oil and are used commercially in butters and in chocolate manufacture. They can be roasted and chopped to decorate desserts. To skin them, bake first in a moderate oven for 15 to 20 minutes. When cool, the skin can be easily removed with your fingers.

Food Content of Filberts (Hazelnuts) (per 100 g): calories, 634; protein, 12.6 g; fat, 62.4 mg; carbohydrate, 16.7 g; fiber, 3.0 g; calcium, 20.9 mg; phosphorus, 337 mg; iron, 3.4 mg; sodium, 2.0 mg; potassium, 454 mg; magnesium, 233 mg; copper, 1.28 mg; manganese, 4.8 mg; zinc, 2.6 mg; vitamin A, 107 IU; vitamin B_1, 0.46 mg; niacin, 0.9 mg; vitamin B_6, 0.5 mg; folic acid, 0.07 mg; pantothenic acid, 0.96 mg; vitamin C, trace.

PEANUTS *(Arachis hypagae)*

Peanuts have been discovered in Peruvian tombs dated 950 B.C. They are also called groundnuts because they grow on long tendrils below the ground. Another name for them is monkey nuts. They are, strictly speaking, legumes, as the shell is the dried pod of the plant. Portuguese explorers took them from Brazil to East Africa during the sixteenth century. Traders fed them to slaves on the sea voyages from Africa to the shores of the United States, where nuts left over were planted to start a major industry. Peanuts are used mainly to make peanut butter, although sesame butter is probably of better food value.

Food Content of Peanuts (per 100 g): calories, 564; protein, 26 g; fat, 47.5 g; carbohydrate, 18.6 g; fiber, 2.4 g; calcium, 69 mg; phosphorus, 401 mg; iron, 2.1 mg; sodium, 5 mg; potassium, 674 mg; magnesium, 175 mg; copper, 0.44 mg; manganese, 1.59 mg; vitamin A, trace; vitamin B_1, 1.14 mg; vitamin B_2, 0.13 mg; niacin, 17.2 mg; biotin, 34 mg; folic acid, 0.1 mg; pantothenic acid, 2.08 mg; vitamin E, 6.5 mg.

PECANS *(Carya illinoensis)*

Pecans—and hickory nuts—are indigenous to America. Pecans are cultivated in Texas and Oklahoma, and in the southeastern United States and are now being exported to Europe. Hickory nuts grow wild in the northern states of the United States. Both were a vital staple food for the American Indians. Pecans are, of course, used in the famous pecan pie; they are also used in nut breads and salads or for decorating kantens and sweets. Pesto sauce can also be made with pecans.

Food Content of Pecans (per 100 g): calories, 687; protein, 9.2 g; fat, 71.2 g; carbohydrate, 14.6 g; fiber, 2.3 g; calcium, 73 mg; phosphorus, 289 mg; iron, 2.4 mg; sodium, trace; potassium, 603 mg; magnesium, 131 mg; copper, 1.05 mg; manganese, 1.42 mg; zinc, 3.0 mg; vitamin A, 130 IU; vitamin B_1, 0.86 mg; vitamin B_2, 0.13 mg; vitamin B_6, 0.169 mg; niacin, 0.9 mg; folic acid, 0.024 mg; pantothenic acid, 1.6 mg; vitamin C, 185 mg.

PINE NUTS *(Pinus pinea)*

The seeds of the stone pine, which is a native of Italy, are packed into the hard, mosaic casing of the pine cone. The trees are now cultivated all around the Mediterranean coast and the nuts are used in many recipes—in Italy, for example, *pesto Genovese* is a popular sauce. They are also chopped and used in stuffings, sweet and sour sauces, and rice bases. In the Middle East they are a popular addition to dolmades. They have a distinctive and pleasant taste but need cooking time to help dissipate the somewhat "turpentine" flavor.

Food Content of Pine Nuts (per 100 g): calories, 642; protein, 13.2 g; fat, 51.1 g; carbohydrate, 20.7 g; fiber, 1.1 g; calcium, 10.7 mg; phosphorus, 610 mg; iron, 5.36 mg; sodium, (–); potassium, (–); vitamin A, 35.7 IU; vitamin B_1, 1.3 mg; vitamin B_2, 0.25 mg; niacin, 4.79 mg; vitamin C, trace.

PISTACHIO NUTS *(Pistacio vera)*

The pistachio is the seed of the fruit from a small tree native to Syria. The Roman epicurian Lucius Bitellus developed a pistachio passion when he was governor there and had large quantities of them shipped back to Rome. From there they were taken to the rest of the known world. The pistachio has been cultivated for thousands of years in Syria, Turkey, Israel, Greece, and Italy and is today grown in California and Texas. It is one of the most popular nuts in America today. It is eaten raw or is mixed with commercial ice creams, used in puddings and cookies, stuffings, sauces, baking, and for sweet dishes. It is sometimes an ingredient of *halva* or *locoum* (Turkish delight). The natural nuts have a delicate green color. The bright red ones are, of course, dyed and usually have refined salt all over them.

Food Content of Pistachio (per 100 g): calories, 587; protein, 13.3 g; fat, 53.5 g; carbohydrate, 18.7 g; fiber, 2.0 g; calcium, 130.7 mg; iron, 7.3 mg; phosphorus, 500 mg; potassium, 967 mg; magnesium, 158 mg; copper, 1.12 mg; vitamin A, 229 IU; vitamin B_1, 0.7 mg; vitamin B_2, (–); niacin, 1.4 mg; folic acid, 0.06 mg; vitamin C, (–).

WALNUTS (Juglans regia)

The walnut tree is also of Middle Eastern origin and was called the Persian Tree by the Greeks who described the nut as *karyon* (*kara* means head) because its convolutions resembled those of the brain. The walnuts grown in the Northern Hemisphere are called English walnuts in America but are known also as French or Italian walnuts in Europe. Black walnuts, which are native to North America, have very hard shells and were stored by the Indians as an important food supply. Walnuts are used as a flavoring or topping in Western cooking. In the Middle East they are pickled or used for making stuffings and sauces. In Italy they are sometimes used to make *pesto*.

Food Content of English Walnuts (per 100 g): calories, 651; protein, 14.8 g; fat, 64 g; carbohydrate, 15.8 g; fiber, 2.1 g; calcium, 99 mg; iron, 3.1 mg; phosphorus, 380 mg; potassium, 450 mg; sodium, 2 mg; magnesium, 131 mg; copper, 1.39 mg; manganese, 1.8 mg; zinc, 2.26 mg; vitamin A, 30 IU; vitamin B_1, 0.33 mg; vitamin B_2, 0.13 mg; niacin, 0.9 mg; vitamin B_6, 0.73 mg; biotin, 37 mg; folic acid, 0.066 mg; pantothenic acid, 0.9 mg; vitamin C, 2 mg; vitamin E, 1.5 mg.

Oils

Most plant foods—vegetables, grains, legumes, nuts, and seeds—contain varying proportions of oil, some more than others. Carrots, for example, have 0.2 grams per 100 grams. Avocado, which is botanically a fruit, has an oil content as high as 16 percent. Brown rice contains 1.8 percent, and soybeans a high 10.3 percent. Nuts and seeds are much higher: walnuts are one of the richest in oil at 64 percent and safflower seeds have 59.5 percent fat. Coconut contains 35 percent fat, 30.4 percent of which is saturated. Most of the oils extracted from plant sources are polyunsaturated but Nan Bronfen recommends using them as little as possible and eating the whole foods instead. Extracted oils are invariably subjected to heat of some kind during processing and are potentially more toxic, and rancid oils can cause a loss of vitamins in the body. It is better generally to sauté vegetables in water, as frying food increases the fat content of your meal and, at extreme temperatures, fat decomposes to produce irritants such as *acrolein*, which can affect skin and mucous membranes. Use oils sparingly for flavor rather than swamping the food with them. Buy them "unrefined" and cold pressed whenever possible and store them in a cool, dark place.

CORN OIL

Corn has been pressed for its oil since the Peruvians began cultivating it many thousands of years ago. It is relatively easy to extract by centrifugal force, and some doctors advise using it externally for skin disorders. It is also a good, general purpose oil for light cooking. It is, however, more yin than most other oils and boils over if used for deep frying (*see* Grains).

Food Content of Corn Oil (per 100 g): calories, 900; protein, (–); fat, 10 g (saturated), 78.6 g (unsaturated); carbohydrate, (–); fiber, (–); calcium, trace; phosphorus, (–); sodium, trace; potassium, (–); zinc, 0.18 mg; vitamin A, trace; vitamin B$_1$, trace; vitamin B$_2$, trace; niacin, trace; vitamin C, trace, vitamin E, 77.8 mg.

OLIVE OIL

Homer and Pliny praised the virtues of olive oil and the Hebrews used it for ancient anointing ceremonies and regarded the olive as a symbol of prosperity. Olives are more easily cold pressed without heat or chemical processing. The first cold pressing produces *virgin* or *Lucca* oil, which may have a greenish tinge and a rich olive scent. Other olive oils are a blend of this oil with hydraulic extractions. Olive oil gives a distinctive flavor to your cooking and makes salads reminiscent of the sunny Mediterranean! It can be combined with an oil such as safflower, which is richer in linoleic acid, for use as a salad oil or cooking medium.

Food Content of Olive Oil (per 100 g): calories, 885; protein, trace; fat, 10.7 g (saturated), 80 g (unsaturated); cholesterol, trace; carbohydrate, trace; fiber, (–); calcium, 0.5 mg; phosphorus, (–); sodium, 0.007 mg; potassium, trace; iron, 0.07 mg; copper, 0.07 mg; zinc, 0.18 mg; vitamin A, (–); vitamin B$_1$, (–); vitamin B$_2$, (–); niacin, (–); vitamin E, 5.1 mg.

PEANUT OIL

Peanut oil is also known as *Arachis* oil or groundnut oil. At present, manufacturers are not obliged to state which extraction methods are used, and the cheaper brands of peanut oil generally use chemical solvents. The oil is then refined, heated, and treated with antioxidants. (*See also* Nuts.)

Food Content of Peanut Oil (per 100g): calories, 885; protein, trace; fat, 10 g (saturated), 78.7 g (unsaturated); cholesterol, trace; carbohydrate, trace; fiber , (–); calcium, trace; phosphorus, (–); sodium, trace; potassium, (–); iron, (–); copper, 0.07 mg; zinc, 0.18 mg; vitamin A, (–); vitamin B$_1$, (–); vitamin B$_2$, (–); niacin, (–); vitamin C, (–); vitamin E, 12.8 mg.

SAFFLOWER OIL

Safflower and sunflower oils are often regarded as interchangeable but are, in fact, quite different, even though both plants are members of the same composital family. The tall thistlelike safflower was cultivated by ancient civilizations along the Nile, and the Arabs have adopted its cultivation. Each safflower seed contains half its weight in oil, which is richer in linoleic acid (up to 80 percent) than any other oil. Sunflower oil is the second richest. The extraction of the safflower oil is difficult, however, because of the hard, shining husk that has to be pressed with powerful hydraulic machines and sometimes chemical solvents are used. The method of pressing applied is not always stipulated on the label. Safflower oil contains up to 75 mg of vitamin E per 100 grams of oil.

Food Content of Safflower Oil (per 100 g): calories, 886; protein, (–); fat, 7.9 g (saturated), 84.3 g (unsaturated); cholesterol, trace; carbohydrate, (–); fiber, (–); calcium, trace; phosphorus, (–); sodium, trace; potassium, (–); iron, trace; copper, (–); zinc, 0.18 mg; vitamin A, trace; vitamin B$_1$, trace; vitamin B$_2$, trace; niacin, trace; vitamin C, trace; vitamin E, 75 mg.

SESAME OIL

Sesame oil has been used for cooking in Africa and the Far East for centuries and is probably one of the best quality oils for general cooking. It is the principal vegetable oil of Mexico and is used as a flavoring in Chinese cooking. As there are no husks to be removed, the extraction of sesame oil can be achieved in a single cold pressing, producing a clear, pale-yellow colored liquid with the advantage that in hot and tropical climates it is not turned rancid by heat. Dark or "toasted" sesame oil is obtained by further pressing of the seeds under hydraulic pressure and is not considered "top grade" oil. It has a heavier, distinctive flavor that can at times enhance the cooking of certain vegetables if used sparingly. Snowpeas are delicious sautéed in a little toasted sesame oil with ginger. (*See also* Seeds.)

Food Content of Sesame Oil (per 100 g): calories, 857; protein, trace; fat, 13.6 g (saturated), 77.9 g (unsaturated); cholesterol, trace; carbohydrate, trace; fiber, (–); calcium, trace; phosphorus, (–); sodium, trace; potassium, (–); iron, (–); zinc, 0.18 mg; vitamin A, (–); vitamin B_1, (–); vitamin B_2, (–); niacin, (–); vitamin C, (–); vitamin E, 56.4 mg.

SUNFLOWER OIL

The sunflower seed is generally second only to the safflower in linoleic acid content. Seeds grown in hot climates contain a lesser proportion than those grown in more moderate areas. Seeds from African plants, for instance, have as little as 20 percent, while certain Russian species can produce up to 70 percent. This linoleic content is considered of medicinal value and is thought to limit the risk of cholesterol deposits in the blood vessels. As with other oils, the less it is processed the better, and it needs to be used in moderation. (*See also* Seeds.)

Food Content of Sunflower Oil (per 100 g): calories, 885; protein, trace; fat, 12.8 g (saturated), 85.7 g (unsaturated); cholesterol, trace; carbohydrate, trace; fiber, (–); calcium, trace; phosphorus, (–); sodium, trace; potassium, (–); iron, (–); vitamin A, (–); vitamin B_1, (–); vitamin B_2, (–); niacin, (–); vitamin C, (–); vitamin E, 9.3 mg.

Okara

This coarse soybean pulp, left over from making *tofu,* can be cooked with vegetables.

Rice

(*See* Grains.)

Rice Syrup

Made from barley malt and rice, it is used as a sweetener. Also sold as "Yinnie syrup," "rice honey," and "rice malt."

Rice Vinegar

(*See* Brown Rice Vinegar.)

Sashimi

This is the Japanese name for raw fish that has been cut into thin strips. It is generally served with a dip made with tamari, water, grated ginger, and daikon or horseradish. The fish can be placed on a finger of soft, pressed rice and decorated with boiled or steamed vegetables and grated daikon. The arrangement, when serving, is very important. Fish to use are boned filet of red snapper, striped bass, tuna, sole, and so forth. Slice diagonally, with a sharp knife, no more than 1/4" thick. (*See also* Sushi.)

Salt–Sea Salt and Rock Salt

Refined table salt is practically pure sodium chloride with sugar, starch, phosphate of lime, potassium iodide, and other substances often added. To the ancient Egyptians and Chinese, salt was a "giver of life" because it preserved food. Salt fish was a standard food for the Greeks; the Romans were skilled at mining it and extracting it from the sea. Salt has become synonymous with good faith and a worthy person is still referred to as the salt of the earth, but even in biblical times, because of taxes levied on salt, it was often adulterated with clay and chalk. There are two types of natural salt: rock (or land) salt, which occurs in veins below the ground, and sea salt, obtained by evaporating sea water. Sea salt has a high iodine content, but rock salt tends to contain less lead and phosphorus because it was formed before people began to pollute the oceans of the world. Crystal salt is mined rock salt or sea salt in large crystal form and is additive free. Salt is yang and can be used in a solution as a disinfectant or gargle. A sea salt compress can be made by roasting salt in a dry skillet for several minutes, placing it in a cotton sack, wrapping it in a towel, and applying it to relieve intestinal or menstrual cramps and muscle stiffness. When using it for cooking, add it only to bring out the flavor of the food, not to make it taste salty. The average diet contains far too much sodium (*see* THE BODY—A LABORATORY—Minerals, Sodium).

Sea Vegetables

Archaeological sites of ten thousand years ago indicate that sea vegetables are possibly the oldest crop known to humans. The ancient Greeks and Romans, however, paid little attention to them as food or medicine. In fact, European use of sea vegetables has been limited. The French have used *kelp* mainly as fertilizer and, in times of war, the potassium from it to make gunpowder. However, today you can buy *laver* from the market stalls in Cardiff and *carrageen,* known as Irish Moss in Ireland. *Dulse* (or *dillisk*) is still eaten in Scotland, and in parts of Alaska dried seaweed is rolled and used as a substitute for chewing tobacco! The Australian coastal Aborigines and the New Zealand Maori used sea plants for food. Seaweeds are an important part of the diet in China, Korea, Southeast Asia, Hawaii, and particularly Japan, where *nori, kombu,* and *wakame* are cultivated. Along the Pacific coast of the United States people eat *ulva,* and the Japanese and Chinese there collect great amounts of laver. In South America, ulva and kelp seaweeds are known as "goiter sticks," a prevention against goiter, which is a common disease in some areas.

Sea vegetables are, in fact, a remarkable source of nourishment, and with recent research they are becoming appreciated for their supply of minerals. According to the Norwegian Institute of Seaweed Research, they can contain some thirteen vitamins, twenty amino acids, and sixty trace elements. They are particularly rich in iodine, iron, and calcium; in vitamin A, the B vitamins, and even vitamins C and D. For macrobiotics they are an essential part of cooking.

Seaweeds are *not* a source of calories and are low in fat. They assist in the digestion of beans when cooked with them, help make superb soups and soup stocks, and they can be roasted and ground to make condiments or used in salads and vegetable dishes.

There is a salad mix available in the United Kingdom made from finely chopped nori, dulse, and sea lettuce (*Ulva lactuca*) that is delicious with noodles (*see* Recipe 66). They are said to have antibiotic qualities, relieve constipation and intestinal and respiratory irritation, promote weight loss, and relieve gout and rheumatism.

Here are some of the chief varieties:

AGAR-AGAR *(Kanten)*

Agar is a gelatin-like substance made from various kinds of red algae. Traditionally, the ribbons of the *gelidium* species were raked and gathered under water to a depth of thirty feet, dried, cleaned, then boiled in huge iron kettles over a wood fire until it congealed. Then it was cut into strips and laid out on bamboo mats in the rice fields during the winter months where it froze at night and melted by day, taking cloudy impurities with it. The flaky, brittle celluloid-like substance was then grated. This was called *Kanten*. Agar-agar flakes, *gracilaria*, are a more recent product, and are generally used for cooking because they are easier to process and have more bonding properties. Agar does not actually dissolve in water, but absorbs it, becomes soft, and swells. When heated to 80°C or more it melts, becomes viscous, and coagulates as it cools. It sets at 25°C to 35°C but does not melt as readily as gelatin, which, by the way, is made by boiling parts of animals, for example, calves feet! Agar also sets firmer—so use it sparingly. (To use Agar *see* Kanten.)

Because few bacteria are able to decompose it, Agar is used commercially as a stabilizer for jams and jellies, as a filler for canned meats, in cosmetics, and as a substrate for bacterial culture.

Food Content of Agar-Agar (per 100 g): calories, (–); protein, 2.3 g; fat, 0.1 g; carbohydrate, 74.6 g ; fiber, (–); calcium, 400 mg; phosphorus, 8 mg; iron, 5 mg; sodium, (–); potassium, (–); vitamin A, (–); vitamin B$_1$, (–); vitamin B$_2$, (–); niacin, (–); vitamin C, (–).

ARAME *(Eisai bicyclis)*

Arame is harvested wild and is wind dried; it may be parboiled, then shredded. It is produced in Japan on the Pacific northeast coast and is eaten when the fronds are young. Another variety grows on the Pacific coast of the United States. Cooked arame may be eaten with a marinade of umeboshi vinegar, tamari, and barley malt. It is generally used in soups, with rice, or with other vegetables. Wash quickly under cold water, then soak in fresh water for 3 to 5 minutes (keep the soaking water).

To cook arame and vegetables:

> 2 cups arame
> 1 teaspoon sesame oil
> 1 medium, sliced onion
> 1 carrot, sliced into matchsticks
> 2 cups soaking water plus 1/2 cup water
> 3 to 4 tablespoons tamari

1. After soaking arame strain off soaking water (and keep). If arame is not already shredded, slice finely.
2 Heat skillet and add oil. Layer on onion, carrot, and then arame. (Do not mix until they are cooked.) Add soaking water plus 1/2 cup more. Reduce heat and cover. Simmer for 10 minutes.

3. Remove cover, add tamari, cover, and cook another 10 minutes.

4. Remove cover, increase heat, and boil off excess liquid.

5. Mix vegetables and arame and serve.

Delicious served with fried tofu!

Food Content of Arame (per 100 g): calories, (–); protein, 7.5 g; fat, 0.1 g; carbohydrate, 60.6 g; fiber, 9.8 g; calcium, 1,170 mg; phosphorus, 150 mg; iron, 12 mg; sodium, (–); potassium, (–); iodine, 98–564 mg; vitamin A, 50 IU; vitamin B_1, 0.20 mg; vitamin B_2, 0.20 mg; niacin, 2.6 mg.

CARRAGEEN or IRISH MOSS *(Chondrus crispus)*

Dried seaweed called *carrageen* has long been a food in Ireland. The name is said to have originated from a village named Carragheen on the coast of Waterford in the south, where Irish moss is gathered and distributed. It is used in folk medicine to treat respiratory disease and was boiled with milk in times of famine. Carrageen is a red algae that is harvested, washed in sea water, and spread on the shore to dry and bleach until it is white or light yellow. Although when packaged carrageen appears to be an unappetizing tangle, the fronds are pretty when washed and soaked. It has a high viscosity in dilute solutions and mixes with various liquids. Consequently it is used commercially as a stabilizer and emulsifier for food processing in ice creams, fruit syrups, sherbets, cheeses, and instant soups. It is also used in the glue, textile, and cosmetic industries. In cooking, carrageen can help thicken soups, stews, and puddings or can be used in jellies and aspics. It can be deep-fried and sautéed with vegetables.

To make a basic jelly:

> 1 cup soaked carrageen
> 5 cups water or vegetable water

1. Soak the carrageen, wash and clean thoroughly. Strain off water and rinse. Discard soaking water.

2. Bring water or vegetable stock (for savory jelly) to a boil. Add carrageen.

3. Simmer for 1/2 hour.

4. Strain off carrageen liquid.

The liquid can be used as base for jellied soups or jelly for fish dishes. The rest of the carrageen can be added to soups or stews.

DULSE *(Palmaria palmatta)*

In Scotland a hundred years ago *dulse tangle* and other sea plants were sold on the streets of Edinburgh. In Ireland, where it is still popular, dulse is called *dillisk* or *crannogh*. It is reddish purple in color and can be eaten raw in salads, or can be steamed or fried. It becomes sticky when boiled and is useful in soups. Because dulse is harvested in the wild and has undergone very little preliminary processing, it is necessary to wash it thoroughly and to remove any tiny shells that may be attached to the surface. If using it for salad, dip in boiling water after washing. Dulse also makes a delicious soup.

Food Content of Dulse (per 100 g): calories (–); protein, (–); fat, 30 g; carbohydrate, (–); fiber, 6.7 g; calcium, 567 mg; phosphorus, 22 mg; iron, 6.3 mg; sodium, 2,088 mg; potassium, 8,071 mg; vitamin A, (–); vitamin B_1, (–); vitamin B_2, (–); niacin, (–); vitamin C, (–).

HIJIKI *(Hizikia)*

This plant is another of the brown algae that preserves well because the alginic acids and fuciodan protect the cell walls from bacteria and fungi. After harvesting it is wind dried and parboiled, which turns it a blackish brown color. The leaflike parts of *hijiki* fall away when it is dried, producing dark, wiry, tangled pieces. Although a native of Japan and Hong Kong, hijiki is grown along the coast of China and in other parts of the world. Hijiki is especially rich in iodine, iron, and calcium.

To prepare hijiki:

>   1 cup hijiki
>   4 cups water
>   1 sliced onion
>   2 tablespoons toasted sesame oil
>   4 tablespoons tamari
>   1/2 cup roasted cashews or pine nuts

1. Before cooking, hijiki needs to be soaked for 10 minutes, which will increase its bulk two or three times. Use 3 cups of water to 1 cup hijiki. Strain off and keep the water.

2. Sauté the onion in the oil, then add the hijiki, stir, and simmer for 10 minutes.

3. Add the soaking water plus another cup and bring to a boil. Simmer for 30 to 40 minutes.

4. Add the tamari and stir.

5. Serve sprinkled with roasted nuts.

(*See also* Recipes 100–102.)

Food Content of Hijiki (per 100 g): calories, (–);protein, 10.1 g; fat, 0.8 g; carbohydrate, 30.6 g; fiber, 16.7 g; calcium, 1,400 mg; phosphorus, 59 mg; iron, 29 mg; iodine, 40 mg; potassium, 14,800 mg; sodium, (–); vitamin A, 150 IU; vitamin B_1, 0.01 mg; vitamin B_2, 0.2 mg; vitamin B_{12}, 0.87 mcg; niacin, 4.6 mg; vitamin C, 0 mg.

KELP *(Laminaria sinclairii)*

The history of kelp—as a fertilizer—in Europe goes back to the twelfth century. In the seventeenth century on the west coast of France certain species of kelp meal from brown algae *Laminarie* and *Fucus* were used to make ash, a source of soda for preparing glass. Kelp, in fact, was an important product during the growth of the Western chemical industry: the potassium from it was needed for chemical fertilizers; the iodine from it for photography after 1811; and kelp ash potassium was in demand to make gunpowder during both World Wars. In Europe *Fucus disticus* is known as bladder wrack or popping wrack, as the ends of the branches often expand to form air bladders. Kelp *(Laminaria sinclairii)* is endemic to the Pacific coast of North America. Like other sea plants, kelp is remarkably rich in calcium. It can be roasted and ground into a powder for use as a condiment but is not usually eaten as a vegetable.

Food Content of Kelp (per 100 g): calories, (–); protein, 5; fat, 1.6 g; carbohydrate, 49.1 g; fiber, 4.4 g; calcium, 1,093 mg; phosphorus, 240 mg; iron, 100 mg; sodium, 3,007 mg; potassium, 5, 273 mg; vitamin A, (–); vitamin B_1, (–); vitamin B_2, (–); niacin, 4(–); vitamin C, (–).

KOMBU *(Luminaria Japonica)*

Eating this sea vegetable went out of fashion in the West years ago, but it is still very popular in Japanese and Chinese cooking. It is a brown algae, and there are more than ten species. It grows in deep waters, and the fronds can be as long as fifteen feet. Its popular flavor is due to the amino acid, *glutamic acid*. This flavor has subsequently been isolated from other sources to make the artificial chemical seasoning *monosodium glutamate*. Kombu is rich in iodine and has long been a curative for goiter in the East. It is used to make soup stocks and broths, and kombu added to beans will help cook them faster, will give them flavor, and will make them easier to digest (*see* Legumes). A pinch of *ground* kombu sprinkled onto grains when soaking and cooking them gives an added flavor—and added minerals. To make the powder, take 6 strips of the brittle, dried seaweed from the packet, cut or tear into 1-inch squares, and whisk briefly in a coffee grinder. Store in a small sealed container.

Before using kombu strips, wash and soak them in a little water for a few moments until soft.

To make soup stock:

> 5 cups water (a little more than you will require for the soup)
> 1 piece of kombu 2" x 1^1/$_2$"

1. Place the kombu in the cold water and heat gently.
2. Just before the water boils remove the kombu, as high temperatures dissolve polysaccharides, which make the soup rather sticky. The same piece of kombu can be used several times, or chop it finely and cook it with vegetables, legumes or soups.

Food Content of Kombu (per 100 g): protein, 7.3 g; fat, 1.1 g; carbohydrate, 51.9 g; fiber, 3.0 g; calcium, 800 mg; phosphorus, 150 mg; sodium, 2,500 mg; potassium, 5,800 mg; iodine, 193 mg; vitamin A, 430 IU; vitamin B$_1$, 0.08 mg; vitamin B$_2$, 0.32 mg; vitamin B$_3$, 1.8 mg; vitamin B$_{12}$, 0.3 mg; vitamin C, 11 mg.

LAVER *(Porphyre laciniata)* and NORI *(Porphyre tenera)*

The Welsh in Pembrokeshire still collect laver at low tide and send it to town to be boiled and processed into "black butter." This can be mixed with oatmeal to make laver bread croquettes or spread on whole wheat bread or toast and a squeeze of lemon added. Laver is of the red algae family and a species of it is greatly popular in Japan where it is cultivated. It is called nori (*porphyre tenera, tenera* meaning soft), and in 1973 the consumption of dried *aakusa nori* amounted to 9.6 billion sheets. The California Pacific Coast also yields large quantities of laver, which is popular with the local Oriental populations. Nori has a multitude of uses and is a fine food. It is as rich in protein as eggs and meat—with only a tiny proportion of fat—and contains practically all vitamins, especially vitamin A (the same amount weight for weight as carrots). It is generally stored in airtight containers to keep it crisp, which helps preserve its considerable vitamin C content. It is also rich in minerals. Dried nori sheets can be roasted, cut, or crumbled to garnish noodles and salads or added to soups and stews. Rice can be wrapped in it or rolled to make a laver "black butter."

Food Content of Nori (per 100 g): protein, 35.6 g; fat, 0.7 g; carbohydrate, 44.3 g; fiber, 4.7 g; calcium, 260 mg; phosphorus, 510 mg; iron, 12 mg; sodium, 60 mg; potassium, 3,800 mg; iodine, 0.5 mg; vitamin A, 11,000 IU; vitamin B$_1$, 0.25 mg; vitamin B$_2$, 1.24 mg; niacin, 10 mg; vitamin B$_{12}$, 13–29 mcg; vitamin C, 20 mg.

WAKAME *(Undaria pinnatifida)*

Wakame has been a popular sea plant in cooking for thousands of years, and in Japan from 1970 to 1971 the per capita consumption of it was about 2 1/2 pounds—more than any other sea vegetable, including nori. Wakame is one of the brown algae cultivated in all parts of Japan today. It also grows on the coasts of Korea and China. After the harvest the *Undaria* blades are hung out to dry, much like laundry, on clotheslines. The midribs *(kuki-wakame)* are prized delicacies. Use in soups, bouillabaisse, marinated dishes, or salads. As with kombu the dry sheets can be whisked briefly in a coffee grinder to make a useful powder for sprinkling on grains when soaking or cooking them or to add to soups. Wakame softens the tough fibers of certain foods and can be cooked with beans. It is an important source of calcium, and the laminine it contains is said to prevent hardening of the arteries and to be effective in preventing hypertension.

Wakame is easy to prepare and the grayish dried-up and wrinkled pieces are quickly restored to a tender and handsome green color by brief washing and then soaking for 3 to 5 minutes. Slice the "leaves" carefully into small pieces and make sure that the hard "midribs" are chopped fine and cooked well.

To cook wakame:

> 2 cups soaked wakame, soaking water saved
> 1 medium, sliced onion
> 1 tablespoon tamari

1. After soaking wakame 3 to 5 minutes, drain off water and set aside. Slice wakame into 1" pieces.
2. Place onions in a pot and cover with wakame. Add enough soaking water to almost cover the seaweed. Bring to a boil.
3. Reduce heat and simmer for 30 minutes, or until wakame is soft.
4. Add tamari and simmer another 10 minutes.

Other vegetables—such as carrots, green peas, etc., or cashew nuts—can be added. If wakame is used for salad, wash, soak, and dip briefly in boiling water.

Food Content of Wakame (per 100 g): protein, 1.2 g; fat, 1.5 g; carbohydrate, 51.4 g; fiber, 3.6 g; calcium, 1,300 mg; phosphorus, 260 mg; iron, 13 mg; sodium, 2,500 mg; potassium, 2,700 mg; vitamin A, 140 IU; vitamin B$_1$, 0.11 mg; vitamin B$_2$, 0.14 mg; vitamin C, 15 mg; iodine, 18 mg.

Seeds

Seeds are the ripened ovules of plants and are rich in vitamins, minerals, protein, and oil. The oil they contain is the chief energy store for the new plant (sesame as high as 49 percent). This oil is often extracted by pressure (cold-pressed) or other methods and is then used for cooking. Seeds and the oil from them need to be stored carefully and used sparingly, as both will turn rancid in a short time. As with nuts, keep them in an airtight container in a cool, dark place. Before using, roast them to release some of the oil and to increase the flavor. They make delicious condiments. Of the oils from seeds, sesame oil is probably the most stable and suitable for daily cooking. Sunflower and safflower oils are also recommended. (*See also* Oils.)

The "spice" seeds from the East and the eastern Mediterranean might be used sparingly sometimes for seasoning.

CARAWAY SEEDS *(Carum carvi)*

Carraway seeds are used in baking, cheese making, savory dishes, and to flavor liqueurs! Related to anise, their pungent, characteristic taste can add "spice" to your cooking.

CORIANDER SEEDS *(Coriandrum sativam)*

This is an annual plant related to parsley from southern Europe and the Middle East. The seeds are dried and roasted and can be used ground or whole. Coriander is one of the main ingredients of curry powder. It is sometimes used in pickles.

FENUGREEK SEEDS *(Trigonella foenum-graceum)*

The name *fenugreek* means "Greek hay," but this seed, native to the Middle East, is featured more in Indian than in Greek cooking. It is recommended by one doctor as a source of choline—which aids in the digestion of fats.

POPPY SEEDS *(Papaver somniferum)*

These are seeds of the opium poppy that is native to the Middle East. Some are yellow and some are bluish black, but they contain no habit-forming alkaloid! They feature in Indian and Jewish cooking and are sprinkled to decorate bread and confectionery and to make cakes and bun fillings such as the Jewish *hamentaschen*. Use sparingly.

PUMPKIN SEEDS *(Curcurbita maxima)*

In China the pumpkin is called the "Emperor of the Garden" and is the symbol of fruitfulness. The word is from *pepon*, the Greek for "cooked in the sun." A native of Asia, the pumpkin is a member of the gourd family. Its seeds, with those of the squash, are one of the most popular types for eating. Roasted with perhaps some tamari they can be sprinkled over vegetables with delicious results! They are reputed to be rich in zinc by some nutritionists, but I can find no figures confirming this. They are richer in iron than any other seed and are high in phosphorus.

 The pumpkin seed is an old herbal treatment for prostate disorders, and modern tests by Dr. W. Devrient in Berlin and Dr. G. Klein in Vienna seem to be confirming its effect on "hormone production, the prostate and bladder" and "its regenerative, invigorative and vitalizing influences." It does, though, have a rather high (46.7 percent) fat content.

Food Content of Pumpkin Seeds (per 100g): calories, 553; protein, 29.0 g; fat, 46.7 g; carbohydrate, 15.0 g; fiber, 1.9 g; calcium, 51 mg; phosphorous, 1,144 mg; iron, 11.2 mg; vitamin A, 190 IU; vitamin B$_1$, 0.24 mg; niacin, 2.4 mg; vitamin C (–).

SAFFLOWER SEEDS *(Carthamus tinctoria)*

Safflower is a tall, thistlelike flower, grown by ancient civilizations along the Nile and down to Ethiopia. The Arabs have adopted its cultivation. The oils of the safflower seeds and sunflower seeds are frequently thought of as interchangeable, but the oil extraction processes can be quite different. (*See also* Oils.) Safflower seed oil is one of the richest in linoleic acid (80 percent); sunflower seed oil 65 percent.

SESAME SEEDS (*Sesamium indicum*)

The sesame is an annual plant native to India and, though mythology, it has come to be regarded in the East as the symbol of immortality. It is one of the world's oldest spices and one of the readiest sources of oil (*see* Oils) and grows plentifully. Until fairly recently, however, it was difficult to harvest because the plant literally throws its seeds to the winds when they are ripe; a new, nonscattering variety has now been produced. The oil can be removed in a single cold-pressing and is good for cooking.

Sesame is harvested the world over. The seeds are a particularly rich source of calcium, iron, protein, vitamins, and minerals. In the West they are baked in bread or are used in cakes and cookies. In the Middle East they are ground into a paste to make tahini (*see* Tahini). The seeds are also used to make "sesame salt" (*see* Gomasio).

Food Content of Sesame Seeds (per 100g): calories, 563; protein, 18.6 g; fat, 49.1 g; carbohydrate, 21.6 g; fiber, 6.3 g; calcium, 1,160 mg; phosphorus, 616 mg; iron, 10.5 mg; sodium, 60 mg; potassium, 725 mg; magnesium, 180 mg; copper, 1.6 mg; vitamin A, 30 IU; vitamin B_1, 0.98 mg; vitamin B_2, 0.24 mg; niacin, 5.4 mg; vitamin C(–).

SUNFLOWER SEEDS (*Helianthus annuus*)

The sunflower has been the mystical symbol of many sunlit, primitive peoples, notably the Incas, who worshiped the sun itself. North Americans grew crops of these flowers for medicinal purposes and used the petals for animal food and dyes. Today even the leaves are being used to treat malaria, and the stalks are burned for use as a fertilizer. The Russians have multimillion-rouble crops of sunflowers.

Sunflower seeds are unusually rich in B complex vitamins and are useful for decorating desserts or vegetables. (*See also* Oils.)

Food Content of Sunflower Seeds (per 100g): calories, 560; protein, 24 g; fat, 47.5 g; carbohydrate, 19.9 g; fiber, 3.8 g; calcium, 120 mg; phosphorous, 837 mg; iron, 7.1 mg; sodium, 30 mg; potassium, 920 mg; manganese, 33.3 mg; copper, 1.97 mg; vitamin A, 50 IU; vitamin B_1, 1.96 mg; vitamin B_2, 0.23 mg; niacin, 5.4 mg; vitamin B_6, 1.25 mg; vitamin C, (–).

Seitan

Seitan is a wheat gluten cooked in tamari, kombu, and ginger. It is best made from hard spring whole-wheat flour. It is very high in protein, calcium, and niacin. This traditional food has a meatlike texture and is eaten in many parts of the world. It can be used in soups and stews, cooked with vegetables or in sukiyaki.

Seitan can be bought commercially or made as follows:

> 5 cups whole wheat flour
> 6 cups water
> 1 kombu strip
> 1/3 cup tamari
> 1 tablespoon ginger juice

1. Place flour in a bowl and mix with enough water to make a bread dough. Knead for 5 minutes.

2. Cover dough with warm water, leave for 5 to 10 minutes, then knead it *in the soaking water* for 2 to 3 minutes. This removes bran and starch, and the water becomes milky. Drain soaking water into a jar and refrigerate for use as thickener for stews and soups.

3. Place the sticky gluten in a large strainer and run cold water over it while you knead it for 2 minutes. Change water to hot and knead another 2 minutes.

4. Repeat this alternating hot and cold water 4 or 5 times. The last rinse is with cold water.

5. Cut the gluten into 2 or 3 chunks. Drop these into 3 cups boiling water and boil until they float to the top (10 minutes).

6. Slice into strips (for sautéing) or cubes (for soup).

7. Place with tamari and ginger juice in a pan with 4 cups of water. Bring to a boil.

8. Add gluten, reduce heat, and simmer, uncovered, for 25 to 40 minutes.

Sesame Butter

(*See* Tahini.)

Sesame Salt

(*See* Gomasio.)

Shiitake Mushrooms

Referred to as "medicinal mushrooms" shiitake are imported dry from Japan and need to be soaked for 15 to 30 minutes before cooking (keep soaking water for soups or stews). They can be obtained fresh in the United States and Europe. The thick, fleshy cap has a smooth, firm texture. The ends of the stalks may need to be trimmed as they can be tough, but the delicate flavor of shiitake is a delicious addition to soups, rice dishes, or sauces. They are a high-protein vegetable. Shiitake tea is made by boiling 2 or 3 mushrooms in water for 15 to 20 minutes. Remove the mushrooms and drink the "tea." It is used to help the discharge of yang from eating too much meat and dairy products, fish, buckwheat, or salt but should be taken only every few days.

Food Content of Shiitake Mushrooms (per 100g): calories, (–); protein, 12.5 g; fat, 1.6 g; carbohydrate, 65.5g ; fiber, 5.5 g; calcium, 30 mg; phosphorous, 80 mg; iron, 5.5 mg; sodium, 30 mg; vitamin A, (–); vitamin B$_1$, 0.05 mg; vitamin B$_2$, 0.03 mg; niacin, 0.5 mg; vitamin C, 20 mg. They are also reputed to contain 2,639 IU of vitamin D.

Shiso *(Perilla frutescens)*

This plant is a member of the mint family. *Shi* means "purple" and *so* means "leaf." Because of its color it is known also as the beefsteak plant. The *shiso* leaves provide the color and flavor in pickling umeboshi plums and also contain *perilla aldehyde*, which is a strong preservative. A condiment sold commercially is made by roasting the leaves from umeboshi production (*see* Umeboshi Vinegar). After roasting, the leaves are ground and can be sprinkled on grains and soups or can be used to flavor rice balls. If obtainable fresh, the purple (yin) *shiso* leaves are useful in salads and as a garnish for soups.

Michio Kushi in *Macrobiotic Home Remedies* says that *shiso* leaves contain chlorophyll, vitamins A, B$_2$, and C; calcium, iron, and phosphorus. They are traditionally used to help the treatment of colds and to calm the nervous system.

Shoyu Sauce

(*See* Tamari.)

Soba

(*See* Noodles.)

Soybeans

(*See* Legumes.)

Soy Sauce

(*See* Tamari.)

Sukiyaki

Sukiyaki is a popular dish in Japanese restaurants and is traditionally cooked at the table, but it can as easily be prepared in the kitchen and served at the table. You can use your cast-iron skillet and the ingredients can consist of vegetables with noodles, seitan, fish, or tofu products (*see* Recipe 179).

Sushi

There are, in fact, several types of sushi, and if you have ever watched the delicate precision and artistry of a good Japanese chef at a sushi bar you have probably tasted *nigirizushi*—a variety of different fish strips, raw or cooked, pressed onto small oval beds of sushi rice with a flavor of horseradish. It is served with fresh, shredded daikon.

Most people's introduction to sushi in a Japanese restaurant is *tekkamaki*—raw tuna fish and sushi rice rolled in a sheet of nori seaweed, and served with ginger and *wasabi* with a soy sauce dip. *Tekka* means "gambling place" and just as the Earl of Sandwich invented that quick "snack" named after him so that he could gamble without interruption, so apparently the Japanese invented *tekkamaki!*

The sushi nori rolls, or *nakizushi*, can have various ingredients wrapped in the rice and nori—fish, daikon or pickles, carrots or other cooked root vegetables, or green vegetables such as cucumber.

Sushi nori rolls are bite-sized, the roll 1" in diameter and the slices 1/2" or so thick. If you make them too large, eating them can be a messy business—but they do make delicious snacks. Be sure you roast the nori sheets so that they stay crisp (*see* Recipe 124).

Tahini and Sesame Butter

These are made from roasted or unroasted seeds. *Tahini* or *tahina* is popular in the Middle East and is the principal ingredient of *halva* and *hummus*. Tahini is prepared from ground, hulled, white seeds and is lighter in appearance. Sesame butter, on the other hand, is made from the unhulled roasted seeds and is darker. The butter is therefore a more complete food. Both are high in oil but can be used for salad dressings, as spreads for breads or rice cakes, as sauces, and as flavoring for soups or in cakes. A spoonful added to rice while cooking gives a delicious nutty flavor to the grain.

Tamari or Shoyu

The word *tamari* is found in Japanese documents as early as 776 c.e. It was the liquid that rose to the surface of soybean *hishio miso* during fermentation. The Japanese characters used for writing the word *tamari* meant "soybean filtering." The liquid from soybean miso kegs was ladled off and heated to stop fermentation. It became popular as a savory seasoning and remains so today.

In 1560 a product known as *tamari-shoyu* became popular. It was made by combining a koji containing soybeans and roasted barley with sea salt and water. A hundred years later shoyu was being produced commercially from equal parts of soybeans and roasted, cracked wheat. By 1670 early traders discovered it and were taking it back to Europe. Dutch traders exported it to France at the request of Louis XIV, who used it at his banquets. From early in the nineteenth century up to and during World War II, the rapid westernization of Japan led to the use of more and more commercial, short-cut methods in the shoyu industry. Stainless steel and concrete tanks began to replace the traditional cedar vats. Today most brands of "soy sauce" are cheap, quick, synthetic products, manufactured in a few days and sold under Chinese brand names. No fermentation time is required, and they are usually prepared with defatted soybean meal and hydrolyzed vegetable protein—even hydrochloric acid is sometimes used! They can be flavored with additives, such as monosodium glutamate, corn syrup, or caramel, and some varieties may contain sodium benzoate or alcohol preservatives. A recent hazard is that the beans used may not be organic but genetically manipulated. So read your labels!

Tamari is the name recently given to soy sauce or shoyu prepared by reputable makers using natural traditional fermentation of soybeans, or soybeans and wheat with sea salt and spring water. It is brewed for up to three years in wooden barrels that have been used and reused over the centuries. Tamari is a rich dark brown and is of a fairly thick consistency. It is obtainable in any good natural food store. The name *tamari* is used to distinguish from the quick, commercial brands.

Tamari or shoyu is used mainly as a condiment to flavor soups, vegetables, cereal and rice dishes, and sauces, or is served with noodles and broths; it is also used for basting, grilling, sautéeing, and boiling. It mixes with brown rice vinegar, umeboshi plums (on fish), wasabi, or with lemon juice for dips. Don't swamp food with it, though. It is very yang. Use a little in the right place!

Food Content of Tamari (per 100g): calories, 68; protein, 5.6 g; fat, 1.3 g; carbohydrate, 9.5 g; fiber, (–); calcium, 82 mg; phosphorus, 104 mg; iron, 4.8 mg; sodium, 8,367 mg; postassium, 457 mg; vitamin A, (–); vitamin B$_1$, 0.02 mg; vitamin B$_2$, 0.25 mg; niacin, 0.4 mg; vitamin C, (–).

Teas

BANCHA TEA

Bancha is sometimes called *three-year tea*. Bancha, in fact, means "three tea," that is, the plant from which it was picked was at least three years old when harvested. Bancha is a good, general purpose drink and will give you a gentle lift at any time of the day. It is prepared like ordinary tea, a teaspoon per person and one for the pot, but it is more economical; boil it for 5 minutes in a stainless steel or enamel pot on the stove. You have only to add water and reboil it to make further supplies. (*See also* Kukicha.)

GENMAICHA

This is a green tea mixed with roasted, puffed rice. It has a unique sweet flavor.

GREEN TEA

All teas, in their numerous forms, come originally from the same plant; various blends derive their different flavors and fragrances from the way the tea leaves (or twigs) are processed and cured. The tea plant was taken from China to India by the English, and Japanese tea also had its origins in China. A priest named Eisai, a Zen Buddhist of the twelfth century, was apparently evangelical in his enthusiasm for tea and attributed to it such benefits as clearness of thinking and longevity. Tea grew well in Japan, where Eisai took it, and it became so popular there that the mystique attached to it, influenced by Zen, became formalized in the practice called *sado,* or the tea ceremony.

Green tea can be harvested at any time of the year. The leaves picked are the young ones, but the later in the season they are picked the less caffeine and tannin they contain. *Green tea should not be boiled.* It needs only to be steeped for several minutes in hot water in a pot. A 1/4 cup of dried tea leaves will provide enough tea for 4 people. The tea need not be dark in color, and the leaves can be steeped 3 or 4 times. It is, of course, not drunk with milk and sugar, but its subtle, bitter taste is good at the end of a meal or with desserts.

KUKICHA

Kukicha means "twig tea" and is made mainly from the twigs of the tea plant, harvested late in the year when the caffeine content is at its lowest level. It is roasted to improve the flavor and to reduce the tannic acid content. The twigs of kukicha have an even lower caffeine content than do those of Bancha. It is probably the most suitable beverage for everyday use. For the preparation of kukicha *see* Bancha Tea.

MUGICHA

Mugicha is tea made from roasted, unhulled barley boiled in water. It is usually sold preroasted and prepackaged in natural food stores, but barley can be roasted in a dry skillet until dark brown. Store in an airtight container.

MU TEA

Mu tea—which one lady journalist thought was our family name for tea with milk—is in fact a blend of some sixteen different herbs. *Mu* means "unique," which Mu tea certainly is. It is a product of George Ohsawa's studies and combines herbs according to their yin and yang properties. Ginseng, one of the most highly regarded Chinese herbs, is one of them. Other herbs included can be peony root, Japanese parsley root, cinnamon, licorice, peach kernels, gingerroot, rhemannia or even mandarin orange peel, atractylis, cloves, montan, and coptis.

This invigorating drink is delicious with a dash of apple juice and is good for the stomach. Mu tea is yang and should not be used regularly or in large quantities. It is usually sold in tea bags, each one making 4 or 5 cups of tea when boiled in water for 10 minutes. The tea bags can be used a second or third time, and the contents can help flavor pastries.

Tekka Miso

The word *tekka* is made from the Chinese characters for metal and fire. This condiment was cooked in a heavy iron pot over low heat. The ingredients used to make tekka are *hatcho miso*, sesame oil, and various roots. They are sautéed over low heat for several hours. It is a popular flavoring sprinkled over rice, deep-fried tofu, and so forth. Tekka is a blackish brown powder said to have medicinal properties. It is rich in iron, is very yang, and is to be used sparingly.

To make fine-textured crumbly tekka miso:

> 2 tablespoons unrefined sesame oil
> 1/4 cup grated carrot
> 1/4 cup grated lotus root
> 1/4 cup grated burdock root
> 2 1/2 teaspoons grated gingerroot
> 1/4 cup black sesame seeds, ground to a paste (or sesame butter)
> 1/4 cup bonito flakes
> 1 cup hatcho miso

1. Heat an iron skillet and coat it with oil.
2. Add the roots, sesame and bonito flakes. Sauté for 5 minutes.
3. Add the miso, stirring well, until the ingredients are mixed evenly.
4. Reduce heat to low and cook gently for 3 to 4 hours. Stir from time to time until the tekka miso is dry, black, and as crumbly as possible.

Makes 2 cups

Food Content of Tekka Miso (per 100g): calories, 249; protein, 9 g; fat, 5.2 g; carbohydrate, 42.8 g; fiber, 2.0 g; calcium, 1.5 mg; phosphorus, 250 mg; iron, 60 mg; sodium, (–); potassium, (–); vitamin A, (–); vitamin B1, 0.10 mg; vitamin B_2, 0.15 mg; niacin, 1.5 mg; vitamin C, (–).

Tempeh

Tempeh is a food popular in Indonesia. It is produced by a natural culture of soybeans and sometimes other legumes, seeds, or grains. The process is very similar to that by which cheese or yogurt is made. Tempeh has a full-bodied, meaty texture and can be used as a main course and substitute for meat—in stews, soups, spreads, sauces, sushis, or sandwiches. It is readily available in the United States. There are even tempeh "burgers" on the market, which are seasoned with tamari, ginger, and other spices, and also deep-fried strips that go well with a touch of French mustard.

The flavor of raw tempeh has been variously described as "nutty," "mushroomy," "yeasty," and "moldy." The taste may, in fact, be one that is acquired. Tempeh, like most raw food, needs seasoning. Try marinating it in tamari, fresh grated ginger, and apple juice. Simmer for about 1½ hours. The protein content of tempeh is a high 19.5 percent, which compares favorably with animal products, but another important nutrient contribution is vitamin B_{12}, which is often lacking in a vegetarian diet. The *rhizopus* mold used in tempeh fermentation produces natural antibiotic agents that are thought to increase the body's resistance to intestinal infection.

Food Content of Tempeh (per 100g): calories, 157; protein, 19.5 g; fat, 7.5 g; carbohydrate, 9.9 g; fiber, 1.4 g;

calcium, 142 mg; phosphorus, 240 mg; sodium, (–); potassium, (–); iron, 5.0 mg; vitamin A, 42 IU; vitamin B$_1$, 0.28 mg; vitamin B$_2$, 0.65 mg; niacin, 2.5 mg; vitamin B$_6$, 830 μ; vitamin B$_{12}$, 3.9 μ; vitamin C, (–).

Tempura

The fish of the famous English favorite "fish and chips" are tempuraed! Sliced vegetables—pumpkin, onion, carrot, parsley—and noodles look quite beautiful after the same treatment. Small pieces of fish, prawns, vegetables, grain patties, tofu, and even fruit slices make a delightful and decorative dish served with rice. The best-quality oil to use for tempura is sesame oil. Corn oil is too yin for deep-frying and will tend to bubble over onto the stove. It is possible to make tempura by shallow-frying, but the results can be untidy.

To make tempura:

> 3/4 cup whole wheat pastry flour
> 1/4 cup cornmeal
> 1/4 cup rice flour
> 1/2 cup fine-ground oatmeal (optional)
> 1 cup cold water
> 1 tablespoon kuzu in 1/2 cup water
> 1/4 teaspoon salt
> Various vegetables, noodles, fish, or prawns (peeled)

1. Mix the dry ingredients and water gradually, stirring until the batter is smooth and creamy. Add kuzu and water. The mixture shouldn't be too runny.

2. Leave the batter to stand in a cool place for at least an hour before using—the longer the better.

3. Place 2 or 3 inches of oil in a pan and heat to 350°F—just before it begins to smoke. Never have the oil too hot. It is ready when a drop of batter placed in it sinks to the bottom and immediately rises to the top.

4. Dip vegetable pieces into the batter and drop into the hot oil. Suitable vegetables for tempura are: carrots sliced diagonally or grated, cauliflower or broccoli florets broken off by hand, Brussels sprouts, sliced or whole mushrooms, pieces of kale, dandelion leaves, parsley, carrot tops, squash, celery in 1½"-pieces, green beans, onion rings or slices, and burdock root. Wash and dry them before dipping them into the batter. Cut them into a variety of shapes. Sliced tofu, small fish pieces, or prawns are also delicious.

5. As the tempura pieces become golden brown, remove them from the oil and drain on paper towels to remove excess oil.

6. Serve with fresh, grated daikon or with grated ginger, tamari, and water to help the digestion of the oil.

Do not reuse the oil for cooking more than 3 or 4 times. Before storing (in a cool, dark place), cook an umeboshi plum in the oil for 10 minutes, then strain off any pieces of batter or food. This will help to preserve it.

Tofu

Tofu is a white bean curd made from soymilk. It is as much part of Oriental culture and cooking as are dairy products in the West. There are some seven different types of tofu in Japan and even more in

China. It is often accused of being "tasteless," but the subtle, gentle flavor of tofu is very adaptable in the kitchen. It can be used for toppings, spreads, dressings, and sauces or is delicious added to soups and stews. It can be pan- or deep-fried to a golden color, broiled, or grilled (with a few drops of tamari added). It will make pie fillings, "tofutti" ices, and dessert toppings and is, of course, a protein booster for grains. It is generally sold in small blocks, water-packed in plastic containers. Tofu can be made at home by using a special tofu box. The white cakes should be kept in water and refrigerated. Change the water every day or so.

Food Content of Tofu (per 100g): calories, 72; protein, 7.8 g; fat, 4.2 g; carbohydrate, 2.4 g; fiber, 0.1 g; calcium, 128 mg; phosphorus, 126 mg; iron, 1.9 mg; sodium, 7 mg; potassium, 42 mg; magnesium, 111 mg; vitamin B$_1$, 0.06 mg; vitamin B$_2$, 0.03 mg; niacin, 0.5 mg.

Udon

(*See* Noodles.)

Umeboshi Plums

The umeboshi blossom, appearing in the cold of late February, rivals the famous cherry for beauty in Japan. *Umeboshi*, "dried plum," was introduced to Japan some thousand years ago and became more popular there than it was in its native China. Its sharp, tart taste is the result of combining yin, green, sour plums with yang, raw salt. The Japanese plum is now a rounder and fatter variety than the original Chinese fruit, which would seem to have a protruding navel as well. The fruit is gathered while it is still green and is packed in vats with raw salt, which draws out a liquid called plum vinegar (*see* Umeboshi Vinegar). The purple *shiso*, or beefsteak, leaves are placed over the plums and the color dyes them a deep red and helps to preserve them. By mid-July, when the rains end and the sun shines, the plums can be spread out, dried, and returned to the umeboshi vinegar.

Umeboshi's flavor is somewhat similar to that of anchovies—without the fishy taste! They are eaten daily in the Orient and are attributed the medicinal properties of helping digestion, settling the stomach, and maintaining the slightly alkaline condition of the blood. They are certainly an invaluable condiment: Their sharp, sour, tangy taste helps to flavor salads. Try slicing one into apple juice, sesame oil, and tamari for a dressing. It is good spread on sweet corn on the cob (with a little olive oil) or placed in the center of a rice ball to preserve it. This preservative factor is due to *perillaldehyde*, which when ingested also helps clear the intestinal tract (*see also* Shiso). Umeboshi and kuzu sauce is a good combination with vegetables, too.

Here are some traditional umeboshi remedies:

UME-SHO-KUZU DRINK

To neutralize acidity, digestive disorders, and diarrhea.

    1 teaspoon kuzu
    1 cup cold water
    1 umeboshi plum
    1 teaspoon tamari

1. Mix kuzu well in the water.

2. Heat the kuzu and water with the umeboshi plum. Bring to a boil.

3. Reduce heat and simmer until transparent. Stir to avoid lumps.

4. Add tamari.

5. Serve hot.

UME-SHO-KUZU AND GINGER

Useful against colds and the flu.

>1 tablespoon fresh ginger juice
>1 teaspoon kuzu
>1 1/2 pints of water, divided
>1 umeboshi plum

1. Mix ginger and kuzu separately in a little cold water.

2. Add these mixtures to the rest of the water, add the umeboshi plum, and bring to a boil.

3. Stir until the liquid becomes transparent.

UME-SHO-BANCHA

Good for headaches caused by too much yin food. Relieves tiredness.

>1 pitted umeboshi plum
>1 cup bancha tea or twig tea
>4 drops tamari

1. Place plum in a cup and pour tea over it.

2. Add tamari.

3. Drink while hot.

Food Content of Umeboshi Plums (per 100g): calories, 17; protein, 0.3 g; fat, 0.8 g; carbohydrate, 3.4 g; fiber, 0.3 g; calcium, 6.1 mg; phosphorous, 26 mg; iron, 2.0 mg; sodium, 9,400 mg; potassium, (–); vitamin A, (–); vitamin B_1, 0.061 mg; vitamin B_2, 0.09 mg; niacin, 0.6 mg; vitamin C, (–).

Umeboshi Vinegar

Plum vinegar is the juice extracted by osmosis from the still green *ume* fruits when they are packed in raw salt for pickling. Its red color is due to the *shiso* leaves placed over the plums (*see* Umeboshi Plums). This highly saline, yet citric solution becomes more and more alkaline with age, and its original, sharp acidity turns increasingly sour. It is sold commercially as umeboshi vinegar or red plum "seasoning" and can make a sharp contribution to salad dressings or sweet and sour sauces. It can be sprinkled sparingly over boiled vegetables and salads or blended with tofu for a sauce.

Wakame

(*See* Sea Vegetables.)

Wasabi

Wasabi is a pale green and fiery horseradish, which is often eaten with Japanese fish dishes (*see* Sushi).

Yannoh

Yannoh is a grain coffee substitute introduced by Georges Ohsawa. It is made from five different grains and beans that are roasted and ground.

Recipes

The recommended balance:

Soups, approximately 5 percent

Grains and Grain Products (breads, pastries, and pancake mixes), 50 percent or more

Vegetables/Sea Vegetables/Salads/Seeds, about 25 percent

Legumes, more or less 10 percent

Sauces, Spreads, and Dips

Animal Products, 5 percent or no more than 10 percent

Desserts, Fruits, and Nuts, a moderate 5 percent

Most of the good cooks I know, when asked for precise recipes, make remarks like, "I used what was left of this ingredient with some from a new packet and enough of the other and a teaspoonful of that." Not much help when you have a publisher to please! But it is the way of cooks and seems to produce the best results.

These recipes simply give an idea of some dishes to cook and the proportions to use. The invention and improvisation is part of the joy of preparing macrobiotic meals.

Approximate oven temperatures for the recipes are indicated in Fahrenheit. Oven temperatures vary with different stoves but the following is a general guide to Fahrenheit and Celsius readings:

LOW OVEN			MEDIUM OVEN			HIGH OVEN			
225°F	275°F	300°F	325°F	350°F	375°F	400°F	425°F	450°F	475°F
107°C	140°C	150°C	170°C	180°C	190°C	200°C	220°C	230°C	240°C

Cup measures are for a full (to the brim) *tea* cup, not a coffee mug or breakfast cup. 1 cup = 1/2 pint or 8 fluid ounces.

Wendy Esko, in *Introducing Macrobiotic Cooking*, says, "Learn to rely on your cookbook as little as possible. The sooner you learn common sense and intuition in cooking the better and more efficient your cooking will become. Once you know the proportions, begin experimenting with different combinations of food. Be creative and artistic . . . instead of using a measuring cup or spoon use the amount that looks right. Trust your senses instead of utensils."

Rice

Soups

In many of these recipes it is suggested you make a soup stock with a strip of kombu in water. It is often quicker and simpler to sprinkle in a pinch of kombu powder when making the soup (*see* INGRE-DIENTS—Kombu).

Using vegetable water:
The less water you use to boil vegetables the better but when you strain it off, save it. Don't pour it down the drain. It is rich in vitamins and useful as a tasty soup stock. It is also delicious to drink with a dash of tamari.

1. Barley Broth

Serves 4 to 6

>   5 cups water or vegetable water
>   2 pinches kombu powder
>   1 cup cooked barley (*see* INGREDIENTS—Grains)
>   1 onion, sliced
>   1 diced carrot
>   1 stalk sliced celery
>   1 cup chopped parsley
>   1 tablespoon soy sauce

1. Bring vegetable water to a boil.

2. Add barley, onion, carrot, celery, and half the parsley. Simmer an hour.

3. Add soy sauce and stir.

4. Garnish with rest of the parsley and serve.

2. Barley, Squash, and Vegetable Soup

Serves 4 to 6

>   2 cups barley
>   2 pinches kombu powder
>   3 to 4 cups water (to soak)
>   10 cups water or vegetable water
>   4 to 6 cups diced winter squash
>   2 medium carrots, sliced
>   2 medium turnips, sliced
>   2 medium parsnips, sliced
>   1 tablespoon corn oil
>   1 tablespoon sesame oil
>   2 tablespoons white shiro miso
>   1 cup hot water
>   1 tablespoon chopped chives or sliced scallion

1. Cover barley with water and soak overnight. Strain off water.

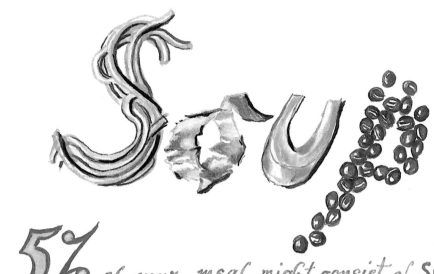

Soup

5% *of your meal might consist of* **SOUP**
WHICH CAN CONTAIN ONE OR ALL OF THE DIFFERENT TYPES
OF FOOD: *grains, legumes, land & sea vegetables, fish etc*
MISO SOUP *can make a complete meal in itself.*

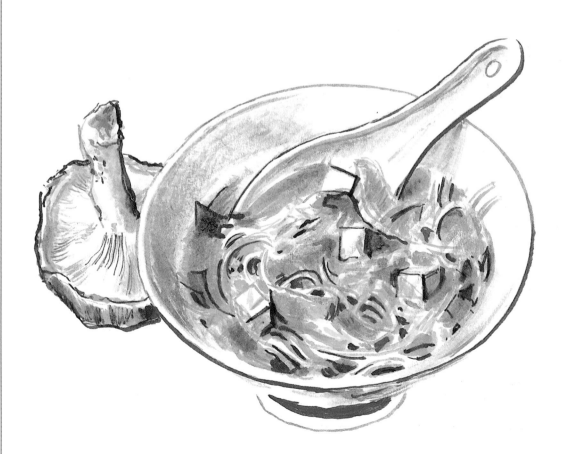

2. Place barley in saucepan with vegetable water and sprinkle on kombu. Bring to a boil, and simmer for 1 hour.

3. Sauté squash and carrots, turnips and parsnips in oil mixture until soft. Let stand until barley is cooked.

4. Add vegetables to barley. Puree two-thirds of the mixture. Mix in the rest of the vegetables.

5. Mix miso in hot water. Add to the pot or to each bowl of soup separately.

6. Decorate with chopped chives or scallion and serve.

3. Beet Soup (Borscht) and Miso

Serves 4

> 2 cups water or vegetable water
> 1 pinch kombu powder
> 1 carrot, finely chopped
> 1 medium onion, finely chopped
> 2 cups beets, finely diced
> 1 cup cabbage, finely shredded
> 1 tablespoon rice vinegar or umeboshi vinegar
> 1 tablespoon shiso miso in 1 cup hot water

1. Bring water to a boil with kombu powder.

2. Add carrot, onion, and beets; cover and simmer gently for 15 minutes.

3. Add cabbage. Simmer another 5 minutes.

4. Mix miso smoothly in water; add vinegar and miso to soup. Bring almost to a boil. Remove from heat.

5. Serve hot or cold with:

> 1/2 cup goat's yogurt
> 1/2 cup grated cucumber
> 1/2 teaspoon shiso condiment or sesame salt

6. Mix the yogurt, grated cucumber, and shiso and add a teaspoon to each bowl of borscht. Sprinkle with your choice of condiment.

4. Bonito, Onion, and Cauliflower Soup

Serves 4

> 2 tablespoons bonito flakes
> 4 cups water or vegetable stock
> 1 large onion, sliced
> 1 tablespoon sesame or corn oil
> 2 cups cauliflower
> 1 tablespoon soy sauce
> 1/2 cup chopped parsley

1. Boil bonito flakes in water or vegetable stock for 5 minutes.

2. Sauté onion in oil until golden brown and soft.

3. Add onion and cauliflower to the bonito water. Simmer 10 minutes.

4. Add soy sauce.

5. Garnish with parsley and serve.

5. Carrageen, Miso, and Pumpkin Soup

Serves 4

> 1/2 cup soaked and washed carrageen
> 4 cups water or vegetable water
> 1 sliced onion
> 1 cup finely diced pumpkin or winter squash (without skin)
> Juice from 1 tablespoon fresh, grated ginger
> 1/2 cup hot water
> 2 teaspoons mugi miso
> 1/2 cup chopped parsley

1. Wash and clean carrageen well.

2. Add to water with the onion and simmer for 20 minutes.

3. Add the pumpkin or squash and ginger juice. Simmer another 20 minutes.

4. Mix mugi miso in water. Add a tablespoon of this to each bowl, pour out the soup, stir, garnish with parsley, and serve.

Wakame or dulse can be used instead of carrageen.

6. Carrageen Jellied Consommé

Serves 4

> 1 cup carrageen, soaked and cleaned
> 1 onion, finely chopped
> 1 teaspoon sesame oil
> 4 1/2 cups water or vegetable water
> 4 teaspoons tamari
> 2 teaspoons umeboshi vinegar (to taste)
> Juice of 1 lemon
> 1/2 cup chopped parsley or chives

1. Braise carrageen and onion in oil for 5 minutes. Add water and simmer for 1/2 hour.

2. Strain off carrageen (keep to use in soups or stews).

3. Add tamari and umeboshi vinegar to the carrageen water.

4. Let set in a bowl or in separate containers. Refrigerate if necessary.

5. Squeeze lemon juice over the consommé and garnish with parsley or chives. Serve cold.

7. Carrot and Bay Leaf (or Orange) Soup

Serves 4

>4 cups water
>1/2 cup soaked wakame, sliced fine
>3 medium carrots, sliced
>1 onion, finely chopped
>2 bay leaves
>2 teaspoons kuzu
>1/2 cup cold water
>1 tablespoon yellow miso
>1/2 cup hot soup
>Chopped parsley or scallions to garnish

1. Bring water to a boil with wakame slices.

2. Add grated carrots, onion, and bay leaves. Simmer 20 minutes.

3. Remove bay leaves. Blend the soup and put back in pot.

4. Dissolve kuzu in cold water and stir into the soup while bringing it almost to a boil. Remove from heat.

5. Take 1/2 cup of the soup mix in the miso, then stir into the soup.

6. Garnish with parsley or scallions. Serve immediately.

Instead of bay leaves, try using juice and grated peel of one small orange when adding the kuzu water.

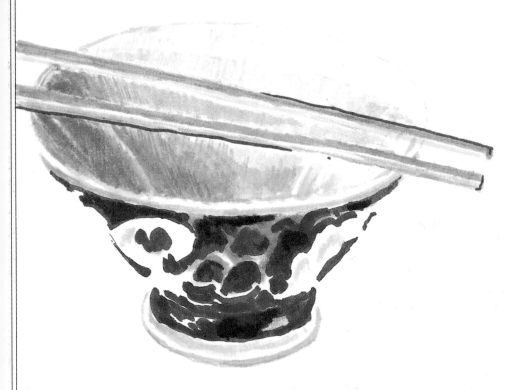

8. Carrot (or Zucchini) and Oat Soup

Serves 4 to 6

6 cups water
1pinch kombu powder
6 medium carrots sliced in 4 pieces or 5 zucchini sliced in 4 pieces
1 cup oat flakes, presoaked (20 minutes)
1 tablespoon white shiro miso
1 cup boiling water
Parsley to garnish

1. Bring water to a boil with kombu and add carrots. Simmer.

2. Add oat flakes, stir, and cook until tender. About 30 minutes. Purée and reheat.

3. Mix white miso in boiling water.

4. Serve soup with parsley and miso on the side to be added to taste.

9. Chickpea Soup with Scallion Garnish

Serves 4

1/4 cup chickpeas
4 cups water
1 large onion
2 strips kombu, 2"x 3" (soaked)
2 teaspoons miso
1 cup hot water
1 cup finely sliced scallion

1. Soak chickpeas overnight in 2 cups water. Discard soaking water. Add Fresh.

2. Slice onion in crescent shapes, and pressure cook with chickpeas, kombu strips, and water for 1 hour (or simmer for 2 hours).

3. Take out kombu strips and chop finely.

4. Mix miso thoroughly in cup of hot water. Add to soup. Heat if necessary, but do not boil.

5. Garnish with scallions and serve.

10. Ginger and Tamari Broth with Tempuraed Parsley

Serves 4

5 cups water or vegetable water
1 teaspoon bonito flakes
1 medium onion, sliced in crescent shapes
2 teaspoons juice from grated ginger
1 tablespoon tamari
1 cup parsley sprigs, tempuraed

1. Bring vegetable water to a boil. Add bonito flakes. Simmer for 2 minutes.

2. Add onion and cook for 10 minutes.

3. Squeeze in ginger juice and add tamari.

4. Serve with tempuraed parsley (*see* Recipe 113).

11. Hijiki and Aduki Soup

Serves 4

    1 cup aduki beans
    4 cups water
    1 strip kombu, 3"x 2"
    1 cup soaked hijiki
    1/2 teaspoon caraway seeds
    1 clove garlic, sliced
    1 tablespoon kuzu
    1/2 cup cold water
    2 teaspoons tamari
    1 scallion, chopped
    1 lemon, sliced

1. Soak aduki beans for an hour. Discard water.

2. Bring aduki and kombu to a boil in the water and simmer for 1 hour. Add water if necessary.

3. Soak the hijiki in water for 10 minutes. Drain and keep the water (about 1 cup). Slice hijiki finely.

4. Place hijiki and water in the aduki beans with caraway seeds and garlic slices. Bring to a boil and simmer another 3/4 hour.

5. Puree 3/4 cup of mixture and return to the pot.

6. Dissolve kuzu in water and add to the soup with tamari, stir well and bring to a boil. Turn off heat. Soup should be creamy thick. Add more water if necessary.

7. Garnish with scallion and serve with lemon slices.

12. Leek Soup with Carrot Flowers

Serves 4

    4 cups water
    1 pinch kombu powder
    4 leaves Chinese cabbage
    1 leek, very finely sliced
    1 carrot, sliced in flowers

1. Add kombu to water. Bring to a boil.

2. Add cabbage and boil 5 minutes, or until soft. Take out. Roll each leaf and slice each roll in half. Place them in the soup bowls.

3. Add leek and carrot to the water and boil 10 minutes.

4. Serve over the cabbage rolls. Garnish with pan-fried mochi squares (as for Miso-Onion Soup, Recipe 17).

13. Lentil Soup

Serves 4 to 6

> 1 large onion, sliced fine
> 1 tablespoon toasted or plain sesame oil
> 6 cups water
> 2 cups lentils (washed)
> 3/4 cup soaked wakame, sliced
> 1 tablespoon genmai (rice) miso, to taste
> 1 sprig parsley or 1 scallion chopped, to garnish

1. Sauté onion in sesame oil for 3 minutes, or until transparent.
2. Add water, lentils, wakame and soaking water to pot. Bring to a boil and simmer for 45 minutes to an hour, or until lentils are soft.
3. Mix miso in 1/2 cup of the soup and stir into the soup to season it.
4. Garnish with parsley or scallion and serve.

14. Miso, Carrot, Scallion, Celery, and Cabbage with Wakame and Tofu

Serves 4

Miso soup can be made using many different recipes, depending on the season and what ingredients are available at the time. There are various types of miso to choose from, each with a distinctive flavor (*see* INGREDIENTS—Miso).

> 4 cups water or vegetable water
> 1/2 cup soaked and finely sliced wakame
> 1/2 cup sliced carrots
> 1/2 cup finely sliced celery
> 1/2 cup sliced savoy cabbage
> 4 sliced scallions
> 1 teaspoon grated, fresh ginger
> 1 tablespoon white shiro miso
> 1/2 cup hot water
> 1 cup tofu, sliced in 1/2" squares

1. Bring vegetable water to a boil with wakame pieces and soaking water.
2. Add vegetables, carrots first, three of the scallions, celery, and cabbage. Simmer for 10 minutes.
3. Mix white shiro miso in the 1/2 cup hot water. Add to the soup with the tofu squares. (If shiro miso is not available, another type will do.)
4. Bring soup *almost* to a boil and turn off heat.
5. Sprinkle the rest of the scallions on top when serving.

The above soup can be made as a meal or snack by adding 2 ounces of whole wheat (udon) noodles or 3/4 cup of cooked, whole grain rice, barley, or oats.

15. Miso, Dulse, and Onion Soup with Tofu

Serves 4

> 2 medium onions
> 3 cups boiling water
> 1 cup washed and chopped dulse
> 2 cups 1/2"-thick slices (2"x 1") tofu
> 2 teaspoons brown rice miso
> 2 scallions
> 1 teaspoon olive oil
> 1 tablespoon sesame salt

1. Slice the onions into thin, even crescent shapes from root to crown.
2. Place in boiling water and simmer, uncovered, until the strong, acid vapors have escaped and the steam begins to smell sweet. The onions will turn translucent in 3 or 4 minutes.
3. Add the chopped dulse and the tofu squares and allow to simmer for 10 minutes. Brush a pan with a little oil, roll tofu in sesame salt and fry gently, until golden brown.
4. Dissolve the miso thoroughly in some of the soup liquid, be sure there are no lumps (use your suribachi). Add 1 tablespoon of mixture to each soup bowl before pouring in soup, and stir.
5. Sprinkle with the finely chopped scallions, top with tofu, and serve.

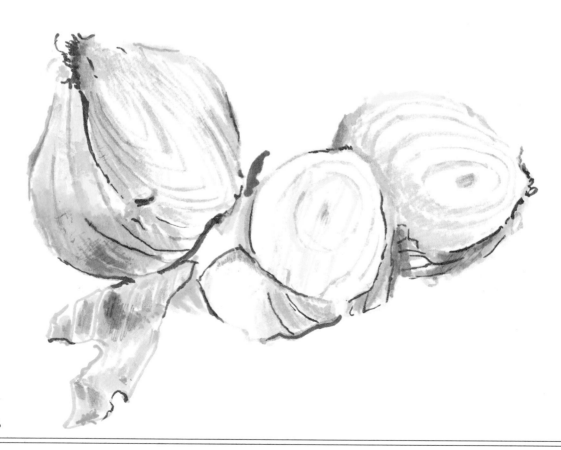

16. Miso, Onion, Pumpkin, Watercress, Dulse, and Soba Noodle Soup

Serves 4

>4 cups water
>1 pinch kombu powder
>1 medium onion, sliced
>1 cup diced pumpkin
>1/2 cup watercress pieces
>1/2 cup washed and finely sliced dulse
>2 ounces soba noodles
>1 tablespoon buckwheat or mugi (barley) miso
>1/2 cup boiling water or the soup liquid
>Chopped parsley or small nori squares as garnish

1. Sprinkle kombu in water and bring to a boil.

2. Drop in onion and allow to boil (uncovered) for 2 minutes.

3. Add pumpkin, watercress, dulse, and noodles. Simmer for 10 minutes.

4. Mix miso well in the 1/2 cup of boiling water or hot soup liquid. Add a tablespoon of this to each bowl before serving.

5. Garnish with chopped parsley or small nori squares.

17. Miso-Onion Soup with Pan-Fried Mochi

Serves 4

>4 cups water
>1 pinch kombu powder
>3 medium onions, sliced
>1 tablespoon mugi miso
>1/2 cup hot water or the soup liquid
>12 1/2" squares of brown mochi rice
>1 tablespoon sesame oil
>1 tablespoon umeboshi vinegar or tamari
>Parsley, as garnish

1. Sprinkle kombu in the water and bring to a boil.

2. Add onions and simmer until very soft (25 to 30 minutes).

3. Puree miso in hot water or soup liquid and add to the onions.

4. Place mochi squares in skillet with a little oil and pan-fry until puffed up and golden brown. Sprinkle with umeboshi vinegar, or tamari, before placing a few in each bowl of soup.

5. Garnish with parsley and serve.

18. Mock Turtle Soup with Batter Croutons

Serves 4

> 5 cups water or vegetable water
> 1 tablespoon bonito flakes
> 1 medium carrot, finely diced
> 1 bay leaf
> 1 tablespoon tamari
> 1/2 sheet nori in 1" squares
> batter croutons
> 1 cup finely chopped parsley

1. Place bonito flakes, carrot and bay leaf in water. Simmer for 20 minutes.

2. Add the tamari and nori squares. Simmer 1 minute.

3. Remove bay leaf and serve with batter croutons and chopped parsley.

BATTER CROUTONS

Serves 4

> 1 tablespoon whole wheat pastry flour
> 1 tablespoon corn flour
> 2 teaspoons kuzu
> Pinch of salt
> 1 cup water (more if needed)
> 1 tablespoon umeboshi vinegar
> 1 tablespoon corn oil

1. Mix flour, kuzu, and salt with water. Stir to make a smooth batter.

2. Let stand for 20 minutes in refrigerator (overnight is better).

3. Add umeboshi vinegar.

4. Brush pan with a little oil, drop "buttons" of batter in, and sauté until golden brown.

5. Dry on paper towels before serving with soup.

19. Mushroom, Carrot, and Noodle Consommé

Serves 4

> 4 cups water or vegetable water
> 1 pinch kombu powder
> 1 small onion, sliced
> 1 medium carrot, sliced
> 6 dried shiitake mushrooms, soaked 20 minutes and sliced or 6 fresh mushrooms, sliced
> 2 teaspoons agar-agar flakes
> 2 cups cooked brown rice udon noodles (*see* INGREDIENTS—Noodles)
> 1/4 cup tamari
> 1 tablespoon mirin or sake (optional) or 1 teaspoon barley malt
> 1/4 of a lemon

1. Place onion and kombu in water and bring to a boil for 3 minutes. Add carrot and shiitake (with soaking water) or fresh mushrooms. Simmer for 25 minutes.

2. Add agar-agar, noodles, tamari, and sake, mirin, or barley malt. Stir over heat for 2 minutes.

3. Leave to set. Serve cold with a squeeze of lemon.

20. Mushroom and Lotus Root Cream Soup

Serves 4

> 3/4 cup finely chopped lotus root
> 6 cups water or vegetable water
> 1 pinch kombu powder
> 1 small onion, chopped
> 6 medium mushrooms, sliced
> 1/2 cup oat or soy milk
> 2 tablespoons tamari
> 2 teaspoons kuzu in 1 cup cold water
> 2 tablespoons chopped chives or parsley

1. If using dried lotus root, soak in 1 cup water until soft enough to chop fine. Add the soaking water to stock.

2. Bring water or stock to a boil with kombu.

3. Add onion and lotus root. Simmer for half an hour.

4. Add mushrooms and boil gently for 10 minutes.

5. Add milk and tamari and blend.

6. Dissolve kuzu in the cold water and stir into the soup. Heat until creamy.

7. Sprinkle with chives or parsley and serve.

21. Onion and Dulse Soup with Tamari

Serves 4

> 1 cup soaked dulse
> 4 cups water or kombu stock (*see* INGREDIENTS—Kombu)
> 4 medium onions, finely sliced
> 2 tablespoons tamari or 1 tablespoon genmai miso, dissolved in 1/2 cup hot water

1. Wash the dulse if necessary and clean off any tiny shells or sand. Chop fine.

2. Bring water to a boil. Put in the onions* and let boil, uncovered, for 2 or 3 minutes.

3. Turn down head to medium-low. Add the dulse and cover.

4. Simmer for 30 minutes.

5. Add the tamari (or miso in water) and stir.

6. Serve with whole wheat bread croutons (*see* Recipe 28).

*Onions can be sautéed first in 2 teaspoons toasted sesame or nut oil.

22. Pumpkin Soup

Serves 4

3 cups pumpkin, peeled and diced
1 pinch kombu powder
4 cups water
1 cup whole wheat bread cubes for croutons (*see Recipe 28*)
2 tablespoons chopped scallions

1. Bring water to a boil with kombu. Add pumpkin to kombu water and cook 1/2 hour. Blend well.

3. Serve with croutons or sprinkle with chopped scallions.

23. Pumpkin and Miso Soup

Serves 4

3 cups water
5 cups pumpkin, peeled and diced
1 teaspoon sunflower oil
1 small onion, chopped
1 clove garlic, crushed (optional)
1 tablespoon ginger juice
1 tablespoon light shiro miso
1/2 cup cold water
2 teaspoons kuzu
2 tablespoons chopped scallions

1. Bring 3 cups of water to a boil and add pumpkin pieces. Simmer for 1/2 hour, or until tender.

2. Brush oil in skillet. Sauté onion and garlic for 5 minutes. Add with ginger juice to pumpkin. Stir.

3. Mix miso in 1/2 cup pumpkin water. Add to cooked pumpkin. Blend mixture.

4. Mix kuzu in cold water and add to the soup. Juice of 1/2 orange can be added with the kuzu. Stir and reheat. Remove from heat before soup boils.

5. Serve with finely chopped scallions on top.

24. Rolled Oats and Celery Soup

Serves 4

6 cups water
Pinch of salt
1 pinch kombu powder
2 cups chopped celery
1 cup rolled oats
Pinch of black pepper

1. Soak oats, salt, and kombu powder in 4 cups water for 30 minutes, then cook another 30 minutes. Add more water if necessary.

2. Add pinch of pepper and celery. Cook 30 more minutes.

3. Puree and reheat before serving.

25. Sea Vegetable Soup

Serves 4

4 cups water
1 tablespoon bonito flakes
1 medium onion, sliced
1/2 cup soaked wakame, sliced in 1/4" squares, water reserved
1 slice 6"x 2" soaked kombu sliced in very small squares
1 sheet nori, cut into 1" squares
1/2 cup dulse, chopped fine
1 tablespoon tamari
2 slices whole wheat bread
1 tablespoon toasted sesame oil

1. Bring water to a boil, add bonito flakes and onion. Simmer for 5 minutes.

2. Add soaking water, wakame, kombu, nori, and dulse. Simmer gently for 10 to 15 minutes.

3. Cut bread into croutons (1/4" squares) and fry in very little oil.

4. Serve croutons in separate bowl to garnish soup.

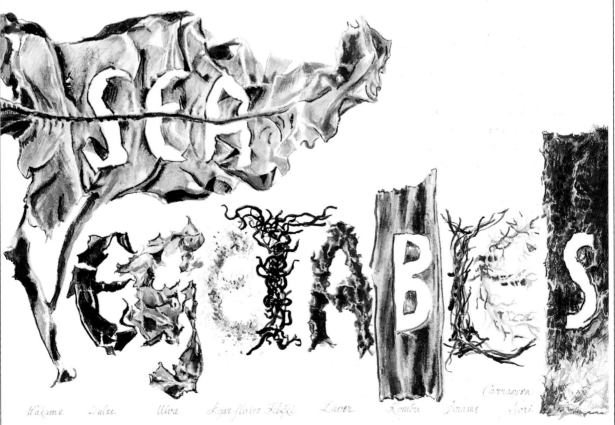

Wakame   Dulse   Ulva   Agar flakes Hijiki   Laver   Kombu   Aname   Nori

26. Shiitake Mushroom and Kombu Broth

Serves 4

> 4 or 5 fresh shiitake mushrooms, sliced (or if dried, soaked for 15 minutes)
> 1 onion, finely sliced
> 1 teaspoon toasted sesame oil
> 5 cups water
> 1 piece kombu, 2"x 3"
> 2 tablespoons tamari

1. If the mushrooms are dried, soak in a cup of water for 15 minutes and use the water for the soup. Remove hard stalk ends.
2. Sauté mushrooms and onion gently in the toasted sesame oil for 5 minutes.
3. Add mushroom soaking water plus 5 cups of water and kombu. Simmer for 30 minutes.
4. Remove kombu and slice into small pieces. Return to soup.
5. Season with the tamari.
6. Decorate with parsley and serve.

27. Seitan and Barley Soup

Serves 4

> 1/2 cup barley
> 4 cups water
> 1 pinch kombu powder
> 1 medium onion, sliced
> 2 carrots, sliced
> 1/2 cup mushrooms, sliced
> 1/4 cup celery, sliced
> 1/2 cup cooked seitan cubes (*see* INGREDIENTS—Seitan)
> 2 tablespoons tamari
> Watercress or chopped scallions, to garnish

1. Wash barley, and soak in water overnight.
2. Add water with kombu powder and boil for 3/4 hour.
3. Add onion, carrots, mushrooms, and celery. Cook 15 minutes.
4. Add seitan cubes. Bring to a boil and simmer for 15 minutes.
5. Add tamari and simmer for 10 minutes.
6. Garnish with watercress or scallions and serve.

28. Watercress Soup

Serves 4

4 cups water
1/2 cup wakame, soaked and sliced
1 small onion, sliced
2 bunches watercress (stalks and leaves), washed well and chopped
Pinch of salt
2 teaspoons kuzu
1/2 cup cold water
Watercress or parsley, chopped, to garnish
Bread croutons

1. Bring water and wakame with soaking water to a boil.
2. Add onion. Simmer gently for 5 minutes.
3. Add watercress and salt and simmer 5 minutes.
4. Blend the soup and return to pan.
5. Mix kuzu in cold water, add to the soup and heat but do not boil; stir carefully.
6. Decorate with watercress or parsley and serve with bread croutons.

BREAD CROUTONS

1 cup whole wheat bread cubes for croutons
1 teaspoon toasted sesame oil
1 teaspoon tamari

1. Brush a skillet with sesame oil and toast the bread cubes gently until golden brown.
2. Sprinkle with tamari but *not* too much on the skillet as tamari will burn.

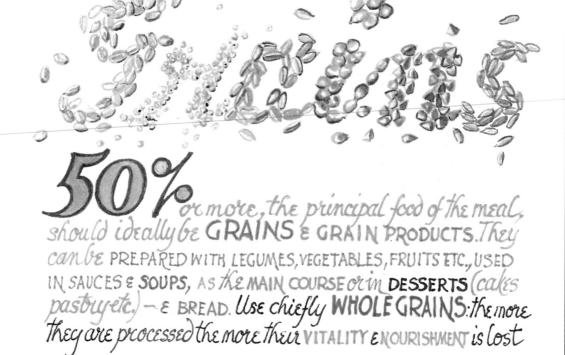

Grains

50% or more, the principal food of the meal, should ideally be **GRAINS** & **GRAIN PRODUCTS**. They can be **PREPARED WITH LEGUMES, VEGETABLES, FRUITS ETC.,** USED IN SAUCES & **SOUPS,** AS THE MAIN COURSE or in **DESSERTS** (cakes pastry etc.) — & BREAD. Use chiefly **WHOLE GRAINS**: the more they are processed the more their VITALITY & NOURISHMENT is lost

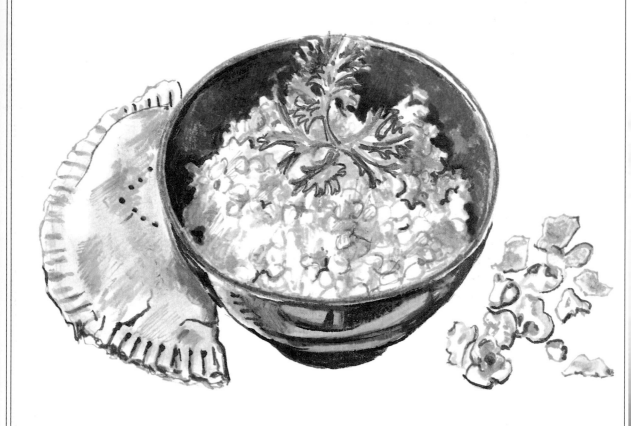

Grains

29. Barley and Burdock Stew

Serves 4

> 1 cup barley
> 4 cups water
> 4 pieces of kombu, each 1" square
> 1/2 cup sliced burdock root (Soak for 10 minutes and discard water.)
> 1 cup water
> 1 cup diced rutabaga
> 1 cup diced celeriac
> Pinch of salt
> Chopped parsley to garnish

1. Soak barley overnight.
2. Add kombu, burdock, and 3 cups of water, bring to a boil and simmer for 45 minutes.
3. Add one cup water, rutabaga, celeriac, burdock, and salt. Stew for 25 minutes.
4. Garnish with parsley and serve.

Barley can be roasted before cooking for a change of flavor.

30. Barley and Vegetable Stew

Serves 4

> 6 dried shiitake mushrooms
> 1 cup water
> 2 cups cooked barley (*see* INGREDIENTS—Grains)
> 1 chopped leek
> 1 carrot, sliced in large pieces
> 1 onion, sliced
> 1 cup water
> 1/2 cup cooked lentils
> 1 tablespoon miso
> 1/2 cup hot water

1. Soak mushrooms in water for 10 minutes and remove stalk ends. Use water for your stew.
2. Place cooked barley in pot and over it the mushrooms, leek, carrot, onion, cooked lentils, and mushroom water, plus 1 extra cup of water.
3. Cook for 1/2 hour over gentle heat until vegetables are tender.
4. Mix miso well in hot water, stir into the stew and just bring to a simmer before serving.

31. Breakfast Muesli Crunch

Serves 8 to 10

> 2 cups oat flakes
> 1 cup wheat flakes or puffed wheat
> 1 cup barley flakes
> 1 cup puffed rice
> 1 teaspoon vanilla (optional)
> 3/4 cup raisins
> 1/2 cup pumpkin seeds
> 1/2 cup sunflower seeds
> 1/2 cup chopped, dried apricots
> 1/2 cup chopped, mixed nuts
> 1 tablespoon sesame salt

1. Mix dry ingredients and vanilla. Place in heavy skillet or pan over low heat. Stir well for 5 to 10 minutes.

2. Allow to cool, and store in air-tight containers.

3. Serve with a teaspoon of rice malt or corn syrup added to each bowl, stewed apples and raisins, or with fruit in season. Pour on apple juice and a dash of oat, rice, or soy milk. Before serving, it is a good idea to soak your muesli for 10 minutes to 1 hour—even overnight.

32. Breakfast Whole Oat Porridge

Whole oats make by far the most nourishing and satisfying morning porridge. Steel-cut oats are quicker to prepare (they cook in 30 minutes). For cooking oats see INGREDIENTS—Grains. Oat porridge can be served hot or cold for breakfast, or as an appetizer or dessert.

SUMMER RECIPE:

Serves 1

> 1 bowl cooked, whole oats
> 1 teaspoon barley malt
> 1/2 tablespoon raisins
> 1 tablespoon Muesli
> 1/4 cup oat milk
> Stewed apples, cinnamon to taste

1. Stir raisins into the cooked oats.

2. Pour barley malt over the top or sprinkle on some Muesli (*see* Recipe 31).

3. Add a dash of oat milk and stewed apples cooked with cinnamon to taste. Serve cold.

WINTER RECIPE:

Serves 1

>   1 tablespoon sauerkraut (in sea salt) or 1 sliced, salt-pickled gherkin (optional)
>   1 bowl hot, cooked oats
>   1/2 teaspoon soy sauce
>   1/2 teaspoon sesame salt or tekka

1. If using sauerkraut or sliced pickles place on top of the cooked oats.

2. Sprinkle soy sauce and sesame salt or tekka.

3. Serve with oat bannocks, hummus, and pressed salad (*see* Recipes 69, 141, 97, and 98).

33. Brown Rice, Aduki Beans, and Vegetables

Serves 2 to 6

A good meal and easily prepared.

>   2 cups cooked short-grained brown rice
>   1 cup cooked aduki beans
>   vegetables

1. For cooking of rice and aduki see INGREDIENTS—Grains; Legumes. Serving them together boosts the protein available (*see* THE BODY—A LABORATORY—Protein Complements).

2. Serve vegetables over the rice and beans.

THE VEGETABLES

The slicing of vegetables is important to the decoration and appearance of the meal. The onions are sliced fine and vertically, the carrots and roots are cut diagonally or sharpened as you would a pencil or are cut in matchsticks or even flowers (see illustrations on pages 28–29, 96, and 156). The greens can also be chopped fine. Use any vegetables in season, except potatoes, tomatoes, or eggplant.

>   1 tablespoon safflower oil
>   1 small burdock root, pencil sliced
>   1 onion, sliced vertically
>   1 carrot, sliced in matchsticks
>   1 small parsnip, sliced
>   2 cabbage leaves, chopped fine or 1 cup bamboo shoots or 6 green beans, sliced
>   4 fresh mushrooms, sliced
>   2 teaspoons kuzu in 1/2 cup cold water
>   1 tablespoon white miso in 1/2 cup hot water

1. Soak burdock root slices for 10 minutes before cooking. Discard water.

2. Heat oil in pan and add burdock root and onion. Sauté gently for 10 minutes, stirring to prevent sticking.

3. Add carrot and parsnip and stir for another 3 minutes.

4. Add cabbage or bamboo shoots or string beans and mushrooms. Stir continually for 5 minutes.

5. Mix kuzu in 1/2 cup cold water and miso in 1/2 cup hot water and pour over vegetables. Add a little boiling water if necessary, heat, and serve over hot rice and aduki beans. Aduki beans may be served as a side dish instead of with the rice.

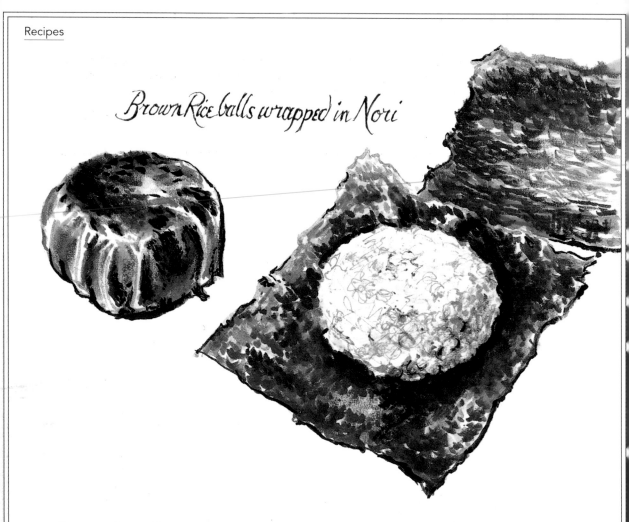

Brown Rice balls wrapped in Nori

34. Brown Rice Croquettes (Rice Balls)

Serves 6 to 8

These are a delicious and practical standby—and they won't stand by all that long! They are made from leftover rice, which needs to be well cooked and soft. They are good for traveling and when proper food is likely to be scarce.

> 3 cups soft cooked, short-grained brown rice
> 1 tablespoon sesame paste (optional)
> 2 umeboshi plums
> 1/2 cup sesame seeds or 1 cup whole wheat bread crumbs
> 1 tablespoon sesame or corn oil

1. If the rice is not soft and sticky you will need to stir in 1/2 cup water and cook gently for 5 minutes, or until the grains hold together. Leave to cool.

2. Add the sesame paste if a nutty flavor is desired.

3. Remove the pits from the plums and slice each into quarters.

4. Wet hands and shape rice into croquettes. Dig a hole in each and place a piece of plum inside— this adds flavor and helps preserve the rice ball when traveling.

5. The surface of the balls should be wet. Roll in sesame seeds or bread crumbs or flour.

6. Rice balls are recommended deep-fried, but you will consume less oil if you wipe the skillet with a little sesame or corn oil and gently pan-fry until golden brown. When cooked, place on paper towels to drain. Serve with salad, parsley sauce, or eat them on their own.

One cup of soft-cooked aduki beans or lentils, chopped parsley, or onion may be mixed with the rice for variety.

These rice balls can also be wrapped in nori sheets instead of frying them. This will keep them fresh when traveling.

> 6 to 8 rice balls
> 3 to 4 sheets nori

1. Roast the nori sheets gently over a flame. They should turn a green-gray color and be crisp.

2. Fold each sheet into quarters and tear neatly into 4 squares.

3. Wrap each rice ball in 1 of the squares. Wet edges to stick the nori to the rice ball.

4. Turn rice ball over and place on a second square, dampen and cover the rice ball with the nori.

35. Brown Rice and Bulgur Croquettes

Serves 4

> 1 cup bulgur
> 1 cup water
> 2 cups soft, cooked brown rice (*see* INGREDIENTS—Grains)
> 2 teaspoons chopped basil
> Pinch of salt
> 1/2 cup chopped parsley
> 1/2 cup flour or 1 cup whole wheat bread crumbs
> 1 teaspoon corn oil

1. Soak bulgur for an hour in a cup of water and steam for 20 minutes.

2. Mix with soft, cooked rice.

3. Add basil, salt, and parsley. Wet hands and shape into croquettes.

4. Roll in flour or bread crumbs.

5. Brush pan with corn oil and sauté gently.

6. Serve with steamed vegetables and Umeboshi Kuzu Sauce (*see* Recipe 163).

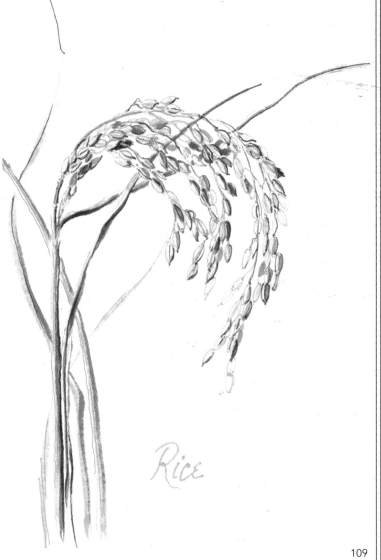

Rice

36. Brown Rice and Chinese-Style Vegetables

Serves 4

3 cups cooked short-grained brown rice (for cooking rice see INGREDIENTS—Grains)
4 shiitake mushrooms
1 large onion, sliced thin
1 large carrot, matchstick-sliced
3 cups shredded cabbage
1/2 cup sliced green or red pepper
3 cups vegetable water
2 cups winter squash, peeled and diced
1 cup snow peas
1 tablespoon kuzu
1/2 cup apple juice
1 teaspoon mirin
2 tablespoons tamari
1 tablespoon roasted sesame seeds, to garnish
Chopped parsley or scallions, to garnish

1. If shiitake mushrooms are dried, soak for 10 minutes in 2 cups water. Slice fine, removing stalk ends, and boil for 15 minutes.

2. Layer onion, carrot, cabbage, pepper, and mushrooms in pot. Add 2 cups of water (and mushroom water). Cover and boil for 5 minutes.

3. Add squash and snow peas. Cover and simmer 5 minutes.

4. Dissolve kuzu in apple juice, add mirin and tamari. Mix with vegetables and stir until mixture thickens.

5. Serve over rice (or noodles) and garnish with sesame seeds and parsley or scallions.

37. Brown Rice and Vegetable Pie

Serves 4 to 6

1 medium onion, chopped fine
4 carrots, sliced fine
1 tablespoon corn oil
2 medium leeks, sliced fine
1/2 cup water
4 cups cooked brown rice
1 cup cooked aduki beans (*see* INGREDIENTS—Aduki)
1/2 cup water
1 clove garlic, crushed
1/2 cup chopped parsley
1 dessertspoon tamari
1 teaspoon light miso in 1/2 cup hot water
2 teaspoons kuzu in 1/2 cup cold water
1 tablespoon tahini
1 teaspoon roasted sesame seeds

1. Preheat oven to 450°F/230°C.

2. Sauté onion and carrots in oil for 5 minutes. Add leeks and sauté, stirring well, for 3 minutes. Add water and bring to a boil.

3. Add vegetables to rice and aduki beans with garlic and parsley. Sprinkle tamari over mixture.

4. Brush a little oil inside pie dish and line dish with pastry (see Recipes 77, 78). Place rice and vegetables in pastry.

5. Mix miso in hot water and kuzu in cold water, pour them into a pan, add tahini, stir, and bring to a boil. Pour this sauce over the vegetables.

6. Cover with pastry, decorate with sesame seeds—press them on top—and bake in preheated oven for 10 minutes. Reduce oven heat to 350° and bake another 25 minutes.

38. Brown Rice Summer Salad

Serves 4 to 6

For taking to the beach in the summer. Keep salad and dressing cool.

  1 Pressed Salad (*see* Recipes 97 and 98)
  3 cups *cold* cooked brown rice (*see* INGREDIENTS—Grains)
  3/4 cup diced apple
  1 cup diced tofu
  1/2 cup seeded raisins
  1/2 cup chopped watercress or parsley
  1/2 cup roasted Brazil nuts or pine nuts
  3/4 cup diced melon or 1/2 cup seedless grapes

1. Mix the ingredients. Place in a container that can be sealed.

2. Keep in a cool place.

Serve with the following dressing:

  1/2 cup apple juice
  2 tablespoons sesame oil
  2 umeboshi plums (pitted & sliced)
  1/2 teaspoon sesame salt
  1/2 teaspoon tamari

1. Mix dressing in a screw-top bottle. Pour dressing over salad immediately before serving.

2. Add more rice if preferred.

39. Buckwheat Burgers

Serves 4

These are made from kasha (*see* INGREDIENTS—Grains).

>1 large onion
>1 tablespoon toasted sesame oil
>1 cup buckwheat, roasted (*see* INGREDIENTS—Grains)
>3 cups water
>2 teaspoons genmai miso
>1 teaspoon light tahini
>3 teaspoons umeboshi vinegar
>1/3 cup hot water
>1/2 cup chopped parsley
>1 cup whole wheat bread crumbs
>1 tablespoon corn or sesame oil

1. Sauté onion in oil for 3 minutes.

2. Add buckwheat and sauté for 5 to 10 minutes, or until golden brown.

3. Add water, bring to a boil and simmer gently for 20 minutes.

4. Turn off heat and let stand, covered, for 10 minutes.

5. Mix miso, tahini, and umeboshi vinegar in the hot water. Pour into the buckwheat, add parsley, and stir well. Cover and let cool. The mixture should be soft and sticky.

6. Wet your hands and shape kasha into croquettes—about 4 to 6.

7. Wet the surface and roll in bread crumbs.

8. Brush skillet with oil and gently sauté "burgers" until brown.

9. Serve with Mochi and Onion Sauce (*see* Recipe 146) or Onion and Squash Sauce (*see* Recipe 151).

40. Buckwheat Kasha with Cabbage and Caraway Tofu Sauce

Serves 4 to 6

>2 cups roasted buckwheat
>4 cups water
>2 tablespoons light tahini
>2 tablespoons umeboshi vinegar

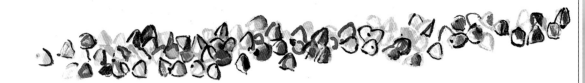

2 teaspoons tamari
1 cup finely chopped scallions
1/2 cup pan-toasted pumpkin seeds

1. Simmer buckwheat gently in water for 20 minutes. Turn off heat and allow to steam 5 minutes. It should be fluffy and soft. Add water if necessary.

2. Mix in tahini, vinegar, tamari, and chopped scallions. Put lid back on and allow to cook for 10 more minutes.

3. Serve with Cabbage and Caraway-Tofu Sauce, sprinkled with pumpkin seeds (*see* Recipe 139).

These can be made into "burgers" if preferred.

41. Buckwheat-Stuffed Squash

Serves 4

1 small summer squash
3 dried shiitake mushrooms, soaked in 1 cup of water (save water) and sliced
1 onion, chopped
1 tablespoon sunflower oil
3/4 cup roasted buckwheat
1 carrot, grated
1 parsnip, grated
1/4 cup chopped parsley
1/2 teaspoon caraway seeds
1 clove garlic, chopped fine
2 tablespoons tahini

1. Preheat oven to 375°F/190°C.

2. Slice squash lengthwise or in 2 1/2" slices and remove seeds. Pour boiling water over and simmer 5 minutes. Drain off water and save.

3. Gently sauté onion for 5 minutes in the oil.

4. Add buckwheat and stir till golden brown (10 minutes).

5. Add carrot, parsnip, shiitake, parsley, caraway seeds, and garlic. Add squash water and shiitake water to make up 3 cups, bring to a boil, stir, and simmer for 10 minutes.

6. Add tahini and stir to make soft stuffing "paste."

7. Fill the squash with stuffing.

8. Bake in preheated oven for an hour.

9. Serve with one of the Béchamel sauce alternatives (*see* Recipe 137).

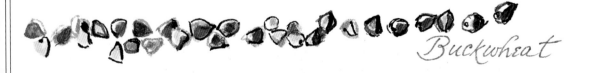

Buckwheat

42. Cabbage Stuffed with Buckwheat with Oatmeal Sauce

Serves 4

4 cabbage leaves
2 cups water
Pinch of salt
1/2 cup chopped onion
1/2 cup diced carrot
1/4 cup diced mushroom
1/4 cup chopped celery
1 tablespoon toasted sesame oil
1 cup roasted buckwheat
1 teaspoon tahini
3 cups water
2 teaspoons genmai miso
1/2 cup hot water
1/2 cup pan-toasted whole wheat bread crumbs

1. Boil cabbage leaves in 2 cups water and salt for 5 or 10 minutes, or until soft. Save water for sauce.

2. Sauté onions, carrots, mushrooms and celery in oil for 5 to 10 minutes.

3. Add buckwheat, tahini, and cabbage water. Bring to a boil, cover, and simmer for 20 to 30 minutes. Remove from heat.

4. Mix miso in hot water and add to mixture. Allow to cool.

5. Cut the hard stem from bottom of cabbage leaves.

6. Shape buckwheat into croquettes with wet hands. Place 1 on each leaf and wrap leaf around it, folding the outer sides toward the center. Roll and fasten with a toothpick. Place in oven.

7. Serve with Oatmeal Sauce (*see* Recipe 150) and sprinkle with bread crumbs.

43. Corn on the Cob with Umeboshi

Serves 4

Delicious served with Maine Lobster.

4 ears of corn
2 cups water
2 umeboshi plums or 2 tablespoons umeboshi vinegar
1 tablespoon olive oil
1 tablespoon tamari

1. Bring water to a boil in a large pot or steamer.

2. Steam or boil corn for 1/2 hour, or until soft.

3. Pit plums and mash with oil and tamari.

4. Spread this mixture smoothly around each ear of corn and serve.

44. Couscous

Serves 4

There are traditional and elaborate ways to prepare couscous that involve considerable time and trouble. This way is quick.

2 cups couscous
4 cups water
1 pinch kombu powder
1 small pinch salt
1 tablespoon olive oil
2 tablespoons raisins
1/2 teaspoon nutmeg (optional)

1. Using a heavy covered pan, bring water to a boil. Add salt, kombu, and oil, and stir.

2. Add couscous and raisins, bring to a boil. Remove from heat. Let stand for 20 minutes.

3. Stir with fork until fluffy before serving.

THE VEGETABLES

2 cups water
2 large onions, sliced in quarters
1/2 cup cooked chickpeas (*see* INGREDIENTS—Legumes)
4 slices summer squash, diced
1 small parsnip, diced
3 carrots, sliced in large pieces
1 leek, sliced in large pieces
1 clove garlic, crushed
1 tablespoon miso
1/2 cup hot water
1 or 2 drops chili pepper (Tabasco) sauce per serving (optional)
1 pinch coriander
1 pinch cumin
1 pinch cinnamon would traditionally be added to vegetables. This is an option but is delicious without.

1. Bring water to a boil, add the onions and simmer for 3 minutes. Add the chickpeas, squash, parsnip, carrots, leek, and garlic and seasoning. Cook for 10 minutes.

2. Mix miso in hot water and add to the sauce.

3. Serve vegetables and sauce over the couscous. Decorate with parsley and add 1 or 2 drops of Tabasco sauce.

45. Couscous or Bulgur Wheat Tabooli Salad

> 3 cups cooked couscous or bulgur wheat (*see Recipe 44*)
> 1 cup finely chopped peeled cucumber
> 1 cup parsley, finely chopped
> 1/2 cup fresh dill, chopped (or fresh mint)
> 1/2 cup raisins
> Pinch of ground coriander (or cumin)
> 1 tablespoon soy sauce
> 2 tablespoons brown rice vinegar
> 1 tablespoon roasted sunflower seeds

1. Mix the cucumber, parsley and dill (or mint) with the couscous (or bulgur wheat) and add raisins.

2. Add coriander (or cumin), soy sauce, and rice vinegar and mix well.

3. Sprinkle with the sunflower seeds.

4. Serve as a cold salad.

46. Five-Colored Rice (Or five shades of beige!)

Serves 4 to 6

> 2 cups short-grained brown rice
> 1/2 cup kombu
> 1/2 cup water
> 6 dried shiitake mushrooms
> 1 cup water
> 1/2 cup dried lotus root
> 1/2 cup water
> 1 cup finely diced fresh burdock root (soaked for 10 minutes)
> 3/4 cup diced tofu
> 1 cup finely diced carrots
> 3/4 cup dried, shredded daikon
> 1/2 cup water

1. Roast rice in a dry skillet until deep golden brown. Stir continually to prevent sticking. When roasted, remove from pan or rice will burn.

2. Soak the kombu for 2 minutes; soak the shiitake and lotus for 10 minutes. Save water. Soak burdock root for 10 minutes and discard water.

3. Place ingredients in pressure cooker in this order: kombu on the bottom, shiitake, tofu, carrots, daikon, burdock, and then lotus. Cover with the rice.

4. Add the soaking water (about 2 1/2 cups) plus 3 more cups.

5. Pressure cook for 45 minutes.

6. Serve with green vegetables or carrots, or mixed vegetables.

47. "Five Element" Vegetable-Millet Pie and Mustard Sauce in Wheatless Crust

Serves 4

1 cup millet
3 cups water
2 pinches salt
1 cup cauliflower pieces
2 teaspoons olive oil
2 medium onions cut in half-moon shapes
2 cups daikon soaked (10 minutes) and sliced in matchsticks
1 cup carrots, sliced diagonally
2 cups broccoli (stems and leaves), sliced diagonally
2 cups chopped kale
2 large scallions, diagonally sliced
1/2 tablespoon tarragon
2 tablespoons fresh, chopped dill
1/2 cup fresh, chopped parsley
2 cooked ears of corn
1 cup broccoli tops, broken small

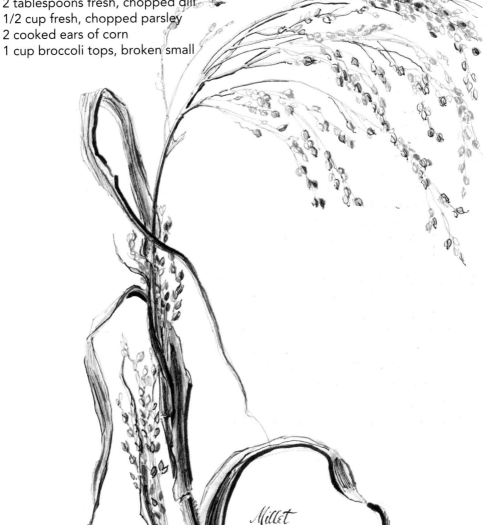

Millet

1. Bring water to a boil in a pan; add millet, salt, and cauliflower.

2. Simmer for 30 minutes. While it is cooking:

3. Heat oil in an iron skillet. Add onion first (sauté for 5 minutes), then daikon, carrots, broccoli stems and leaves, kale, scallions, tarragon, dil, and parsley.

4. Stir well over medium heat for 10 minutes.

5. Remove corn from the cobs.

6. Remove millet and cauliflower from heat and mash the mixture.

7. Add millet and cauliflower, corn kernels, and broccoli tops to vegetable mixture.

MUSTARD SAUCE

> 1 3/4 cups water
> 1 teaspoon kuzu
> 2 teaspoons arrowroot
> 2 teaspoons natural (Dijon) mustard
> 1 tablespoon umeboshi paste or 3 umeboshi plums, pitted and mashed
> 2 tablespoons tamari

1. Mix kuzu and arrowroot in cold vegetable water.

2. Add mustard, umeboshi, and tamari.

3. Heat, stirring well, until the mixture thickens (boil for 3 minutes).

4. Pour the sauce over the vegetable and millet mixture and mix in well.

5. Press Wheatless Pastry (*see* Recipe 82) into a 9" pie dish and spread vegetable-millet and sauce mixture in it.

6. Bake in preheated 375°F/190°C oven for 35 minutes.

48. Fried Rice and Shiitake with Leeks, Chinese Cabbage, and Parsley

Serves 4

> 1 tablespoon corn or sesame oil
> 1 cup cooked shiitake mushrooms, dried or fresh, sliced
> 3 cups boiled brown rice
> 1 tablespoon tamari

1. Oil pan and sauté mushrooms.

2. Add rice and stir-fry 5 to 10 minutes.

3. Sprinkle in tamari.

4. Stir and serve with vegetable below.

THE VEGETABLES

> 1 leek, sliced diagonally
> 1 medium carrot, sliced in matchsticks
> 1/4 Chinese cabbage, cut lengthwise then finely sliced
> 1 teaspoon toasted sesame oil
> Pinch of salt

1 teaspoon kuzu
1 cup water
1/2 cup chopped parsley

1. Sauté leek, carrot, and cabbage in oil and salt until soft, 5 to 10 minutes.

2. Mix kuzu in water and pour over vegetables. Bring to a boil.

3. Sprinkle with parsley and serve with rice.

49. Millet-Aduki Croquettes

Serves 4

2 cups soft, cooked millet (*see* INGREDIENTS—Grains)
2 cups cooked aduki beans (*see* INGREDIENTS—Legumes)
1 carrot, diced
1 cup diced scallions
Pinch of salt
2 1/2 cups whole wheat bread crumbs
1 teaspoon sesame oil

1. Millet should be well cooked, moist, and soft. Beans should also be cooked very soft but not too wet. Mix well together.

2. Sauté carrot and scallions in a little water with salt, for 10 minutes.

3. Mix ingredients, wet hands, and shape croquettes.

4. Roll in whole wheat bread crumbs.

5. Sauté gently in a pan brushed with oil.

6. Serve with Fresh Dill Sauce (*see* Recipe 140) or Onion and Squash Sauce (*see* Recipe 151).

50. Millet-Arame Croquettes

Makes 4 to 6

1 medium onion, chopped
2 teaspoons sesame oil
2 cups soft, cooked millet (*see* INGREDIENTS—Grains)
1 cup cooked arame, chopped fine (*see* INGREDIENTS—Sea Vegetables)
1/2 cup raisins
1 tablespoon soy sauce
1 1/2 cups bread crumbs
1 tablespoon corn oil

1. Heat oil in pan. Add onion. Stir for 3 to 4 minutes.

2. Add millet, arame, raisins, and soy sauce. The millet should be soft. Stir well. Allow to cool.

3. Wet hands and shape into 4 to 6 croquettes.

4. Roll in bread crumbs and sauté in a little corn oil.

5. Garnish with parsley and serve with Lemon Sauce (*see* Recipe 143).

51. Millet and Cauliflower Mash

Serves 4

>1 teaspoon sesame oil
>1 cup millet
>1 1/2 cups cauliflower florets
>1 pinch salt
>1 pinch kombu powder
>3 1/2 cups water

1. Heat oil in a pan with a lid. Add millet and sauté 3 to 4 minutes.
2. Add cauliflower, salt, kombu, and water. Bring to a boil.
3. Simmer, covered, for 30 minutes. Let stand 15 minutes.
4. Mash with a wooden spoon and serve with vegetables (*see* Recipe 53).

52. Millet and Vegetables

Serves 4 to 6

>1 onion, diced
>1 tablespoon toasted sesame oil
>1 small carrot, diced
>2 cups millet (washed)
>6 to 8 cups boiling water
>1 cup fresh green peas
>Pinch of sea salt
>1/2 cup chopped parsley

1. Brush sesame oil over the bottom of a pan. Sauté onion for 2 to 3 minutes.
2. Add carrot. Sauté another 5 minutes.
3. Add millet and sauté 2 or 3 minutes, stir to avoid burning.
4. Add boiling water and sea salt and bring to a boil. Cover and reduce heat. Simmer for 30 minutes. The more water you add, the softer the millet will be. If you prefer it dry, add only 6 cups water.
5. Add the peas and cook another 10 minutes.
6. Stir in parsley and serve with vegetables (*see* Recipe 53).

This mixture can also be used to make croquettes: roll in bread crumbs.

53. Millet and Baked Parsnips with Vegetables

Serves 4

> 1 onion, finely sliced
> Pinch of salt
> 2 cups millet
> 4 cups water
> 1/2 cup chopped parsley

1. Sauté onion in 1/2 cup water and salt for 10 minutes.

2. Add millet and stir for 5 minutes.

3. Add the rest of the water and salt and bring to a boil. Simmer for 30 minutes, or until water has evaporated.

4. Sprinkle with parsley and serve with vegetables.

THE VEGETABLES

> 2 parsnips, sliced lengthwise
> 1/2 teaspoon sesame oil
> Pinch of salt
> 1/4 small cabbage, shredded
> 2 cups diced pumpkin
> 1/2 cup washed ulva, sliced
> 2 cups sliced cauliflower
> 1 tablespoon roasted pumpkin seeds

1. Preheat oven to 350°F/180°C.

2. Sprinkle parsnips with salt and brush with oil. Bake for 1/2 hour.

3. Steam cabbage, pumpkin, ulva, and cauliflower for 10 minutes.

4. Serve vegetables, garnished with pumpkin seeds, around millet.

54. Mochi and Vegetable Casserole

Serves 4 to 6

> 6 shiitake mushrooms, sliced
> 1 onion, sliced
> 1 pinch kombu powder or salt
> 1 tablespoon sesame oil
> 1/2 head cabbage, chopped fine
> 2 carrots, sliced diagonally
> 2 cups mochi in 1" squares (*see* INGREDIENTS—Mochi)
> 2 tablespoons tamari

1. If shiitake mushrooms are dried, soak for 15 minutes (save water) and then slice. Remove stalk ends.

2. Sauté onion, shiitake, and kombu in oil for 5 minutes.

3. Add cabbage and carrots, cover, and simmer for 10 minutes.

4. Pan-fry mochi squares for 5 minutes, until they puff up and are golden brown.

5. Place mochi on top of vegetables, sprinkle with tamari, and serve with rice.

55. Noodles with Radish and Scallions

Serves 4

> 1/4 pound green tea soba noodles
> 2 cups vegetable water
> 1 cup chopped scallions
> 1 cup grated daikon
> 1 teaspoon sesame oil
> 2 teaspoons kuzu
> 1 cup cold water
> 1 tablespoon umeboshi vinegar
> 2 teaspoons tamari

1. Cook the noodles in water (*see* INGREDIENTS—Noodles).

2. Sauté scallions and daikon in teaspoon of oil (3 minutes).

3. Mix kuzu in cold water and add to vegetables. Gently stir and bring almost to a boil.

4. Add umeboshi vinegar and tamari. Serve over noodles.

56. Oat and Rice Patties with Parsley and Onion

Serves 4 to 6

Use boiled whole oats left over from breakfast.

> 1 medium onion, chopped
> 1/2 cup water
> Pinch of salt
> 2 cups soft, cooked short-grained brown rice
> 2 cups soft, cooked whole oats (*see* INGREDIENTS—Grains)
> 1/2 cup chopped parsley
> 1 cup whole wheat flour

1. Braise the onion in water and salt for a few minutes.

2. Add onion to rice and oats and mix in parsley. Mixture should be soft enough to roll into patties. You need to wet your hands to do this.

3. Roll in flour or bread crumbs.

4. Brush pan with oil and place over moderate heat. Gently sauté the patties until golden brown.

5. Serve with Umeboshi-Kuzu Vegetables (*see* Recipe 127) or Mochi and Onion Sauce (*see* Recipe 146).

57. Polenta (Wet or Grilled) with Vegetables

Serves 4 to 6

> 1 1/2 cups whole grain polenta (cornmeal)
> 6 cups water
> 1 pinch sea salt
> 1 tablespoon olive oil
> 2 teaspoons tahini
> 1 1/2 tablespoon umeboshi vinegar or 1/2 cup grated Pecorino or Parmesan cheese

1. Mix polenta and sea salt with 2 cups of cold water and the oil.
2. Bring the rest of the water to a boil.
3. Place polenta mix in a large pan and pour on the hot water gently, stirring constantly to avoid lumps.
4. Cook over the lowest heat for 25 minutes, stirring to prevent sticking. It is cooked when it is thick and falling from the sides of the pan.
5. This is *wet* polenta. Stir in oil, tahini, and umeboshi (or cheese), and serve with:

>1 small zucchini, sliced, or
>3 slices of summer squash (diced)
>2 sliced shallots
>2 large mushrooms
>1 pinch kombu powder or sea salt
>1 tablespoon olive oil
>2 teaspoons miso
>1/2 cup hot water
>1/2 cup cold water
>1 teaspoon kuzu

1. Stir-fry the vegetables in oil.
2. Mix miso in hot water. Mix kuzu in cold water, add to the vegetables, and stir. Heat and serve as sauce over the hot polenta.

For *grilled* polenta: While still hot, place on a plate brushed with oil, spread the mixture 1/2" thick. When cold, cut into slices, wipe with oil, and grill or fry for 3 minutes on either side. Serve with steamed or boiled asparagus, broccoli, or French beans, and sprinkle fine slices of Pecorino Romano or Parmesan.

58. Rice, Avocado, and Corn Salad

Serves 4

For a hot day.

>3 cups cooked brown rice (*see* INGREDIENTS—Grains)
>1 avocado
>2 ears of corn, cooked
>2 salt-pickled cucumbers, diced
>1/2 cup cashew nuts, roasted
>1 onion, finely chopped
>1 teaspoon lemon juice
>1 teaspoon olive oil
>1 teaspoon brown rice vinegar
>1 teaspoon tamari
>4 young lettuce leaves, washed

1. Peel and pit avocado, then slice and mash in with the rice.
2. Remove corn from the cob and add to the mixture.
3. Add cucumbers, cashews, and chopped onion.
4. Mix juice, oil, vinegar, and tamari and dress the salad.
5. Serve chilled over a bed of lettuce.

59. Rice and Bean Croquettes with Mochi Sauce

Serves 4

> 1 cup water
> Pinch of salt
> 1 small onion, finely chopped
> 1 small carrot, finely diced
> 2 cups cooked, short-grained brown rice
> 1 cup cooked black turtle beans (or aduki)
> 1 large umeboshi plum, sliced into six sections
> 3 cups whole wheat bread crumbs
> 2 teaspoons unrefined sesame oil

1. Bring water to a boil and add salt, onion, and carrot. Simmer for 10 minutes, or until carrot and onion are soft.
2. Rice and beans need to be well cooked and soft (*see* INGREDIENTS—Grains; Legumes). Add these to the mixture and stir. Let cool.
3. Wet your hands and from the mixture make six croquettes. Place a piece of umeboshi plum in each. Roll in bread crumbs.
4. Brush oil onto a heavy pan over moderate heat. Add the croquettes. Cook until golden brown, turning occasionally.
5. Serve with Mochi and Onion or Pesto Sauce (*see* Recipes 146 and 152).

60. Rice and Oat Cakes with Onion and Celery

Serves 3 to 4

> 1 cup soft, cooked whole oats
> 2 cups soft, cooked short-grained rice (*see* INGREDIENTS—Grains)
> 1/2 cup water
> 1 large onion, chopped
> 1 clove garlic, chopped
> 2 stalks of stringed celery, finely chopped
> 1 cup chopped parsley
> 1/2 sheet nori pieces, finely cut
> 1 heaping tablespoon light miso mixed in 1/2 cup water
> 2 cups bread crumbs
> 2 tablespoons sesame oil

1. Mix the oats and rice in a bowl.
2. Heat water in pan and add onion and garlic. Stir and braise for 3 minutes.
3. Add celery or parsley and the nori pieces. Stir and cook for 3 minutes. Stir in miso.
4. Mix vegetables with rice and oats. Add 2 tablespoons bread crumbs.
5. Wet hands and make rice cakes—6 to 8—from the mixture.
6. Roll them in bread crumbs and pan-fry until golden brown.

61. Seitan Parcels

Serves 4

Seitan is a very useful wheat protein food, similar to meat in texture (for making it see INGREDI-ENTS—Seitan). It can be bought ready-made, marinated in tamari and ginger, in natural food stores.

> 6 slices of seitan, each about 1 1/2" square
> 3/4 cup pencil-shaved burdock
> 1 tablespoon toasted sesame oil
> 1 cup diagonally cut celery
> 1 teaspoon, fresh, dry, brown mustard
> 2 teaspoons rice vinegar or apple juice
> 1/2 cup water
> 1 tablespoon tamari
> 1 teaspoon grated ginger
> 1 tablespoon sesame or safflower oil

1. Slice a "pocket" in each seitan piece.
2. Soak burdock for 10 minutes before cooking. Discard water.
3. Heat oil in pan. Add burdock and sauté for 10 minutes.
4. Add celery and cook another 5 minutes.
5. Mix mustard in rice vinegar or apple juice and add to the vegetables with tamari and ginger.
6. Place stuffing into seitan pieces.
7. Sauté pockets gently (add a little more oil to pan if needed) and serve with grains and vegetables.

62. Seitan and Vegetable Casserole

Serves 4

> 1 teaspoon sesame oil
> 1 teaspoon corn oil
> 1 cup sliced and soaked (10 minutes) burdock root, discard water
> 1 cup sliced daikon
> 1 large carrot, sliced
> 1 small leek, chopped
> 1 cup sliced fresh mushrooms
> 1 1/2 cups marinated seitan pieces (*see* INGREDIENTS—Seitan)
> 3/4 cup bancha (or kukicha) tea
> 2 teaspoons tamari
> 2 teaspoons kuzu
> 1/2 cup cold water

1. Heat oils in pan. Add burdock and sauté gently for 5 minutes.
2. Add daikon and sauté another 4 minutes.
3. Add carrot and leek and simmer for 10 minutes.
4. Add mushrooms, seitan, tea, and tamari.
5. Dissolve kuzu in cold water and add to thicken the stew.
6. Serve with noodles or rice.

63. Soba Noodles with Tofu "Alfredo" Sauce

Serves 4

>3 cups tofu
>4 cups boiling water
>1 tablespoon white shiro miso
>1 teaspoon basil
>2 teaspoons olive oil
>1 medium leek, finely chopped
>2 medium onions, finely chopped
>4 mushrooms, sliced fine

1. Place tofu in boiling water to blanch it.
2. Remove tofu (keep water), and place in blender with miso, basil, and enough of the blanching water to blend to a creamy texture.
3. Heat the olive oil in a pan, add leek, onions, and mushrooms and sauté for 15 minutes, or until soft.
4. Add tofu cream to the vegetables, heat, and stir well. Serve as a sauce for hot soba noodles (*see* INGREDIENTS—Noodles) and steamed green vegetables.

64. Stuffed Grape Leaves (Dolmades)

Makes 12

>12 fresh grape leaves
>1 1/2 cups water
>1 teaspoon salt

1. Bring water to a boil and add salt. Cook grape leaves in it for 4 minutes and keep the water to make the stuffing.
2. Cut out the lower, hard portion of each center stem.

THE STUFFING

>1 tablespoon olive oil
>1 medium onion, chopped
>2 cups soft, cooked, short-grained brown rice (*see* INGREDIENTS—Grains)
>1 tablespoon currants
>1 tablespoon roasted pine nuts
>1 clove garlic, crushed
>2 tablespoons fresh, chopped parsley
>1/2 teaspoon ground cinnamon
>1 teaspoon grated lemon peel
>1 cup grape leaf water
>3 umeboshi plums, sliced
>Juice of 1/2 lemon
>1 tablespoon tamari

1. Heat oil in pan, add onion and sauté until transparent (3 minutes).
2. Add rice and stir in currants, pine nuts, garlic, parsley, cinnamon, tamari, and lemon peel.

3. Add water from grape leaves. Bring to a boil, stir and simmer for 10 minutes. Add a little more water if necessary.

4. Lay out the grape leaves and place a teaspoon or so of filling in the center of each. Push in a piece of umeboshi plum. Roll the leaf from the bottom over the filling and tuck in the sides as you do so.

5. Arrange the rolled leaves in a steamer with about 3 cups water in the pan. Cover pot and steam gently for 45 minutes over low heat. Be sure leaves are tender.

6. When dolmades are cold, sprinkle with lemon juice and serve. (Keep your steam water for stock.)

65. Sushi with Carrot, Spinach, and Omelet

Serves 4 to 6

> 4 cups soft, short-grained, cooked brown rice (*see* INGREDIENTS—Grains)
> 4 tablespoons umeboshi vinegar
> 1 tablespoon corn or malt syrup
> 1 carrot, sliced in 1/4" wide strips
> 2 dozen spinach leaves
> 2 cups water
> 3 tablespoons tamari
> 2 eggs
> 2 tablespoons tamari
> 1/4 cup vegetable water (from spinach)
> 4 sheets nori
> 1 teaspoon fresh lemon juice or ginger juice

1. Mix soft rice with umeboshi vinegar and corn or malt syrup.

2. Sauté carrot strips in 1/2 tablespoon of the oil over low heat until soft (10 minutes). Let cool.

3. Boil or steam spinach until soft. Strain and keep water. Cool and squeeze into a long, flat shape. Slice into long strips. Sprinkle with 1 tablespoon of the tamari.

4. Mix eggs, the remaining tamari, and 1/2 cup of spinach water. Using the rest of the oil, cook omelet over medium heat. Fold omelet 4 times to make a long shape. Cool and slice into strips.

5. Roast the nori sheets over low flame. They will become a greenish color. Place one sheet on a sushi mat and spread the rice over it. The rice should be spread to about 1/2" from the side edges of the nori sheet and 1" from the top and bottom edges.

6. About 1 1/2" from the bottom edge make a "trench," and place strips of carrot, spinach, and omelet across it.

7. Roll the sushi in the mat as though making a large cigarette. Keep it firm, even and smooth. Wet the edge with lemon juice or ginger juice to stick the nori together.

8. Use a sharp knife to slice the roll to make smaller "sushi" rolls.

(Tofu strips may be used instead of omelet. The tofu is fried and garnished with ginger juice and tamari.) (*See also* INGREDIENTS—Sushi.)

66. Udon (Brown Rice) Noodles with Mushroom Sea-Salad Sauce

There is a sea-salad packaged in the United Kingdom made from finely chopped nori, dulse, and sea lettuce (*ulva lactuca*).

Serves 4

>8 ounces udon brown rice noodles
>1/2 cup sea salad *or*
>1 sheet nori, cut very small
>1 tablespoon dulse, chopped fine
>1 tablespoon sea lettuce (*ulva lactuca*) or arame, chopped fine
>1/2 cup water
>1/4 clove garlic
>1 tablespoon olive oil
>1 medium onion, finely sliced
>6 medium mushrooms, sliced
>2 teaspoons kuzu
>2 teaspoons tamari

1. Bring noodles to a boil and cook over a low flame for 10 to 15 minutes.

2. Soak sea-salad mixture in water for 2 to 3 minutes.

3. Wipe skillet with garlic, heat oil, braise onion for 3 minutes on gentle flame, add mushrooms, and cook another 5 minutes.

4. Strain sea salad (keep water), mix with mushrooms and onion, stir for 2 minutes.

5. Mix kuzu in soaking water, add more water if needed. Stir in with mushrooms and sea salad with tamari, heat and stir until sauce thickens. Do not let boil.

6. Drain noodles. Rinse briefly in cold running water, heat and stir in with salad and mushrooms. Good with broccoli and pan-toasted pumpkin seeds.

67. Udon (Wheat) Noodles and Vegetable Salad

Serves 4

>8 ounces udon noodles
>1 cup sliced cauliflower
>1 cup diced celeriac
>1 cup diced rutabaga
>1 cup broccoli florets
>1 cup red radish, sliced
>1 cup water
>1/2 cup rice vinegar
>1 tablespoon soy sauce
>2 teaspoons kuzu
>3/4 cup water
>1/2 cup pumpkin seeds, roasted in the oven or in a pan

1. Boil noodles in water. (For cooking noodles *see* INGREDIENTS—Noodles.)

2. Strain and rinse in cold water.

3. Boil cauliflower, celeriac, rutabaga, broccoli, and radish in 1 cup water for 2 to 3 minutes.

4. Add rice vinegar and soy sauce.

5. Mix kuzu in cold water. Add to vegetables and bring to a boil. Pour vegetable mixture over the noodles. Decorate with pumpkin seeds and serve.

This recipe also can be made with soba (buckwheat) brown rice udon or chasoba (green tea and buckwheat) noodles.

68. Whole Wheat Spaghetti and Tofu-Parsley Sauce

Serves 4

> 8 ounces whole wheat spaghetti or udon noodles
> 2 cups boiling water
> 1 teaspoon olive oil
> Pinch of salt

1. Preheat oven to 250°F/120°C.

2. Add spaghetti or noodles to boiling water, salt, and oil. Stir well.

3. Boil for 10 minutes, by which time water should be absorbed.

4. Stand (covered) to steam in preheated oven for 10 minutes before serving with:

TOFU-PARSLEY SAUCE:

> 1/2 cup chopped parsley
> 1 teaspoon basil, chopped fine
> 1 teaspoon sunflower oil
> 1 tablespoon rice vinegar
> 1 teaspoon ground pine nuts
> 1/2 teaspoon kuzu
> 3/4 cup water
> 1 cup oat milk
> 1 1/2 cups finely diced tofu

1. Sauté parsley and basil in oil for 2 minutes.

2. Add rice vinegar and pine nuts.

3. Mix kuzu in water, add tofu, and blend.

4. Mix ingredients in a pan and, stirring well, bring to a boil.

5. Serve over the noodles.

Breads, Pastries, and Pancake Mixes

69. Bannocks or Oatcakes

A treat for breakfast.

> 1/2 cup fine ground oatmeal
> 1/2 cup medium ground oatmeal
> 1 tablespoon whole wheat flour
> 1 tablespoon rice flour
> 1 tablespoon corn flour
> 1/2 tablespoon sesame oil
> 1 pinch of salt
> 1/2 cup water (more or less as needed)
> 1/4 cup sesame seeds

1. Mix oatmeals, flours, and sesame seeds with salt and knead in oil.
2. Add just enough water to make a smooth dough—but not too wet. Add more flour if needed. Roll dough into a tube shape 2 1/2" in diameter. Cut into 3/4"-thick, round slices.
3. Sprinkle flour onto a plate and, using your palm, press the slices (each side) into flour. They should then be round biscuit shapes, about 1/2" thick.
4. Toast them on a medium-hot griddle or pan. Turn them until each side is golden (about 10 minutes).
5. Using a sharp, wet serrated knife, slice each cake through the middle to make 2, half as thick. Toast the uncooked surfaces and serve hot.

Delicious with hummus, nori spread, and pressed salad. Also with tahini and sugarless marmalade. (As bannocks are best when fresh, use as much as you need, seal the rest, and keep in a cool place. Will keep a day or so.)

70. Bread with Buckwheat, Chestnut, Whole Wheat, and Rye Flours

Makes 1 loaf

Bread can be made by using various combinations of grain flours. Experiment!

> 2 cups whole wheat flour
> 2 cups rye flour
> 2 cups buckwheat flour
> 2 cups chestnut flour
> 1 tablespoon sea salt
> 3 tablespoons corn and sesame oil mix
> 3 1/4 cups water

1. Mix flours.
2. Mix in salt and add oil carefully. Knead oil in well.
3. Add water gradually and work the mixture thoroughly with your hands, breaking up any lumps. Dough shouldn't be wet.

4. Knead for 10 minutes.

5. Cover dough with a damp cloth and leave in a warm, dry place such as a 95°F/35°C oven. Allow to rise for 24 hours.

6. Knead again for about 10 minutes and place in oiled bread pans to rise for another 4 hours in oven or warm cabinet.

7. Cut a simple crisscross design on the top surface and bake in preheated 325°/170° oven for 45 minutes. For even cooking, place a pan of water in the oven while baking the bread.

If making whole wheat bread, use 8 cups whole wheat flour.

71. Bread with Corn, Rye, and Whole Wheat Flours

Makes 1 loaf

>2 cups whole wheat pastry flour
>1 1/2 cups corn flour
>1 cup rye flour
>1 teaspoon baking powder
>1/2 teaspoon salt
>4 tablespoons oil (sesame and corn mix)
>2 cups organic soy milk
>1/3 cup maple syrup

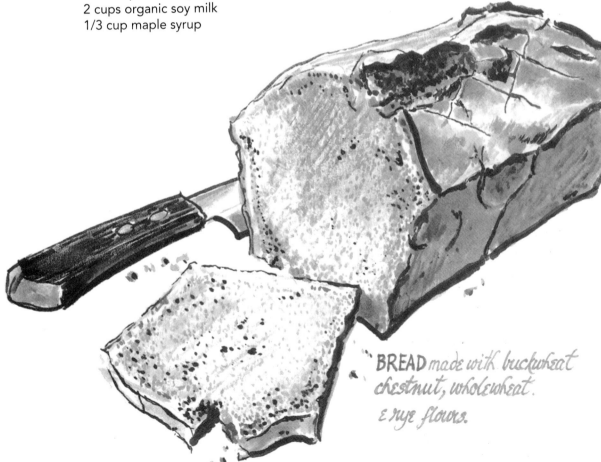

BREAD *made with buckwheat chestnut, wholewheat. & rye flours.*

1. Preheat oven at 350°F/180°C)

2. Mix flours, baking powder, and salt and drop in the oil.

3. Add soy milk and maple syrup and stir thoroughly.

4. Wipe a bread pan with oil and sprinkle with a little corn flour before placing dough in it.

5. Bake in preheated oven for 45 minutes.

72. Bread of Five Grains

Makes 2 loaves

>   4 cups whole wheat flour
>   2 cups rye flour
>   2 cups oat flour
>   1 cup millet flour
>   1 tablespoon sea salt
>   2/3 cup mixed sesame and corn oil
>   3 cups water

1. Mix flours.

2. Mix in salt and pour in oil carefully. Knead oil in well.

3. Gradually add water, working mixture thoroughly with your hands. Do not allow dough to become too wet.

4. Knead dough for 10 to 15 minutes.

5. Cover dough with a damp cloth and leave in a warm, dry place such as a 95°F/35°C oven for 24 hours.

6. Knead another 10 minutes. Place in oiled pans to rise for 4 more hours.

7. Preheat oven to 325°F/170°C. Cut crisscross pattern on top and bake for 45 minutes.

73. Bread Using Sourdough and Onion

Makes 1 loaf

You will need to make a sourdough starter first.

STARTER

>   1 tablespoon dry yeast
>   2 1/2 cups warm water
>   2 1/2 cups whole wheat pastry flour
>   2 tablespoons barley malt or rice syrup

1. Mix ingredients in a jar, and cover with a mesh cloth (several layers of cheesecloth), then seal with a rubber band and leave for 5 days in a warm, dry place.

2. Uncover daily and stir the mixture.

3. After 5 days the starter begins to ferment and will need to be refrigerated.

4. Each time you use some of your starter to make bread, add flour and water. Stir it each day and keep refrigerated.

BREAD:

    1 cup rye flour
    1 cup whole wheat pastry flour
    1 cup millet flour
    1 teaspoon sea salt
    2/3 cup sourdough starter
    2 cups water
    3 medium onions, sliced in crescents
    2 teaspoons corn and sesame oil mix
    1 teaspoon roasted sesame (or caraway) seeds

1. Combine flours and salt and stir well with hands. To make dough, add starter and water. If mixture is too wet, add more whole wheat flour.

2. Cover with a damp cloth and leave in a warm, dry place such as a 95°F/35°C oven for 24 hours to rise.

3. Sauté onions in corn-sesame oil for 5 to 6 minutes and pan-fry sesame (or caraway) seeds until golden brown.

4. Add onions and most of the seeds to dough and shape into a loaf. Leave in oven another 2 1/2 hours to rise.

5. Sprinkle and press in the rest of the seeds on top of loaf. Bake in preheated 325°F/170°C oven for 55 minutes.

This bread can be made using olive oil and 12 black, salt-marinated olives.

74. Buckwheat Pancake Mix

    1/2 cup buckwheat flour
    1/2 cup whole wheat pastry flour
    Pinch of salt
    2 teaspoons kuzu
    1/2 cup rice or oat milk
    1/2 cup cold mineral water (or iced water)
    1 tablespoon safflower/sunflower oil

1. Pour flours in mixing bowl with salt, add milk. Mix kuzu in water and stir in with a fork. Refrigerate for 1/2 hour.

2. Wipe a cast-iron skillet with oil, pour some of the mixture into the center of the hot pan, spreading it to make a *thin* layer of pancake. Turn, cook until golden brown, and serve.

These pancakes can be filled with sweet (*see* Recipe 195) or savory filling. If sweet filling is to be used, add 1/2 teaspoon cinnamon to the mixture.

75. Fruit Pie Crust

> 1 1/2 cups cooked millet
> 1 cup roasted rolled oats
> 1 tablespoon rice or barley malt syrup
> 1 teaspoon miso mixed in 1/4 cup hot water
> 2 tablespoons seeded raisins
> 1 teaspoon soya oil

1. Mix millet and rolled oats.

2. Add syrup and miso mixed in water and raisins. Stir well.

3. Wipe pie pan with oil, press pastry in, and place fruit on top (see Recipe 190).

76. Oatmeal Crust

> 3 cups rolled oats
> 1 1/2 cups whole wheat pastry flour
> 1/2 teaspoon sea salt
> 2 to 3 tablespoons corn oil
> 2 cups water

1. Preheat oven to 375°F/190°C.

2. Mix oats, flour and salt.

3. Add oil and mix.

4. Add water to form a thick batter.

5. Spread batter on an oiled baking sheet or pie pan and bake in preheated oven for 10 minutes.

6. Remove from oven and place fruit or filling on crust and bake again at same heat for 25 to 30 minutes (see Recipes 190, 194, 223).

77. Pastry Pie Crust (for sweet or savory pastries)

Always use cold utensils and keep your hands cold when making pastry.

> 3 cups whole wheat pastry flour
> Pinch of sea salt
> 1/2 teaspoon cinnamon for sweet pastry
> 1/2 cup safflower oil
> 1/2 cup water or 1/2 cup apple juice for sweet pastry (more or less)

1. Mix flour and salt in a bowl. Add cinnamon if desired.

2. Gently pour in oil and mix quickly with your hands or a spoon.

3. Add water, gradually stirring to make dough. Be sure it is *not too wet;* if it is, add more flour.

4. Let stand 1/2 hour before baking.

It can be kept in the refrigerator if you wish to use it later.

78. Pastry Pie Crust 2

>1 cup corn flour
>2 cups whole wheat flour
>Pinch of sea salt
>1/4 cup corn oil and toasted sesame oil
>1 cup water (more or less as needed)

1. Mix flours and salt in a bowl.

2. Gently pour in oil, and mix quickly with your hands or a spoon.

3. Add water gradually, using enough to make a dough that's not too wet. Knead well.

79. Pizza Pastry Pie Crust 3

>2 cups whole wheat flour
>Pinch of salt
>1/2 teaspoon curry powder
>2 tablespoons sesame or corn oil
>1 cup cold water (more or less as needed)

1. Preheat oven to 350°F/180°C.

2. Mix flour, salt, and curry powder in a bowl.

3. Knead in the oil quickly, and gradually add water to make a dough that's not too wet. Let stand 1/2 hour.

4. Sprinkle board with flour and roll out dough.

5. Oil a pie pan and press the pastry in it.

6. Place in preheated oven for 15 minutes to precook the pastry. Use lower oven rack to avoid scorching the top edge.

7. Cover with Aduki Pizza mixture (*see* Recipe 130) and top with sauce (*see* Recipes 137 and 147).

80. Pancakes for Béchamel Vegetable Sauce

Serves 4

>3/4 cup whole wheat pastry flour
>1/2 cup rice flour
>1/4 cup corn flour
>Pinch of salt
>1 cup cold rice or organic soy milk
>1 cup cold water
>2 teaspoons kuzu or
>1 free-range egg
>1 tablespoon sesame oil

1. Mix the kuzu in water, add 1 tablespoon of sesame oil, and the other ingredients, and stir to a thin creamy consistency and let stand in a cool place for at least 1 hour.

2. Brush a little oil on skillet. Heat gently—it should not be too hot. (To test the heat of your skillet, let a few drops of water fall on it. If the water stays and boils the surface is not hot enough: if it vanishes quickly it is too hot. The water should bounce and sputter.)

3. Drop in the pancake mixture. Pancakes should not be too thick. (*See* Recipe 111 for sauce.)

When making dessert pancakes add 1 tablespoon corn or rice malt syrup.

81. Tofu Pie Crust

> 3 cups whole wheat pastry flour
> 1 cup cornmeal
> Pinch of salt
> 1/4 teaspoon cinnamon
> 3 tablespoons corn oil and sesame oil
> 1 1/2 cups water (more or less as needed)

1. Preheat oven to 350°F/180°C.
2. Mix flour, cornmeal, salt, and cinnamon in a bowl. Gently pour in oil mixture.
3. Add water gradually to make a dough. Knead for 8 minutes.
4. Roll out and place on the bottom of a shallow ovenproof dish. Bake in preheated oven for 30 minutes.
5. Add Tofu Filling (*see* Recipe 223).

82. Wheatless Pastry

> 1 cup rye flour
> 1 cup brown rice flour
> 1 cup cornmeal
> 1/3 teaspoon salt
> 1/4 cup mixed corn oil and sesame oil
> 2/3 cup water

1. Mix dry ingredients. Sprinkle in oil and stir well.
2. Mix in water to make dough. Roll out and press into pie pan.
3. Spread with Vegetable-Millet Filling and Mustard Sauce. (*See* Recipe 47 for filling and baking directions.)

83. Whole Wheat Unleavened Bread

Makes 1 loaf

> 6 cups whole wheat flour
> 1 teaspoon sea salt
> 1/2 cup sesame seeds
> 3 cups water
> 1/2 cup goat yogurt (optional)

1. Mix flour, salt and sesame seeds.
2. Add water gradually then yogurt to make a smooth, not too wet, dough.
3. Knead this 200 times. Sprinkle flour on kneading surface if necessary.
4. Wrap dough in a damp cloth and let stand in a warm, dry place, such as a 95°F/35°C oven, for 10 to 12 hours. Knead another 100 times.
5. Oil your bread pan and place dough in it. Sprinkle a teaspoon of sesame seeds on top and press in gently. Slice lines across the top with a sharp knife. Let rise for 1 hour in pan.
6. Preheat oven to 450°/320°C. Bake for 15 minutes, reduce heat to 350° F/180°C and continue baking for 45 minutes. Use lower oven rack.

This bread can be made without being kneaded. It is delicious served with Tahini, Ginger, and Scallion Miso Spread (*see* Recipe 156) or tahini and raisins.

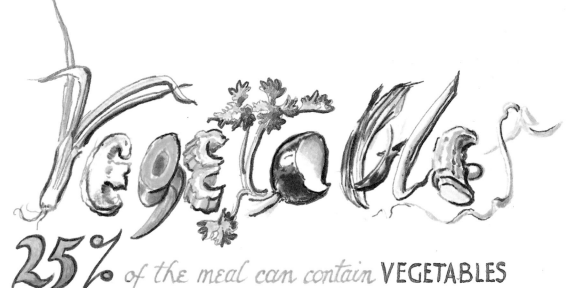

Vegetables

25% of the meal can contain VEGETABLES

THEY CAN BE USED IN SOUPS, AS SIDE DISHES, COOKED WITH THE MAIN GRAIN OR SERVED AS SALADS. *They are usually cooked:* sauteed in a **LITTLE** *oil or water, boiled, baked or steamed.*

5% can be salad   5% SEA VEGETABLES

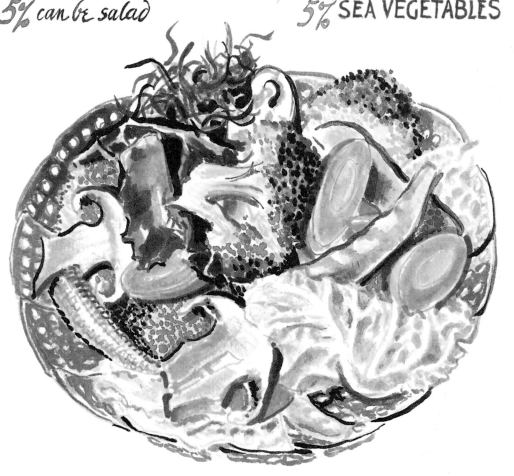

Vegetables

84. Arame and Caraway Seeds

Side dish for 4

>1 cup dried arame
>2 cups water
>1 tablespoon safflower oil
>1 slice onion
>1 teaspoon caraway seeds
>1/2 cup water
>2 tablespoons tamari
>1 tablespoon roasted pumpkin seeds

1. Soak arame in water for 1 or 2 minutes. Remove and keep water.
2. Heat oil in a pan. Sauté onion for 2 minutes. Add arame and caraway seeds and stir for 5 minutes. Pour in soaking water with 1/2 cup more water and bring to a boil.
3. Simmer covered for 30 minutes over low heat.
4. Add tamari, remove cover, and steam off rest of water.
5. Decorate with pumpkin seeds and serve as a side dish.

85. Arame with Onions, Pumpkin, and Roasted Sesame Seeds

Side dish for 4

>1 cup arame
>1 1/2 cups water
>1 tablespoon toasted sesame oil
>2 small onions, sliced
>1 cup diced pumpkin (peeled)
>1 tablespoon tamari
>1 cup water
>1 tablespoon roasted sesame seeds

1. Soak the arame in water for 2 minutes and strain (keep water).
2. Heat sesame oil in a pan. Sauté onions until golden brown.
3. Add arame and stir. Sauté for 5 minutes.
4. Add soaking water plus 1 cup water and tamari, bring to a boil and simmer, covered, for 15 minutes.
5. Add pumpkin, uncover, and boil to remove excess water (10 minutes).
6. Garnish with sesame seeds and serve.

86. Avocado with Sauerkraut Dressing

Serves 2

>1 avocado
>1 tablespoon sauerkraut (see Recipe 115)

1 tablespoon sesame oil
2 tablespoons apple juice
Juice of half a lemon
1 teaspoon chopped parsley or chopped scallion

1. Cut avocado in half, remove pit, and fill each half with sauerkraut.

2. Mix sesame oil, apple juice, and lemon juice and pour over the sauerkraut.

3. Decorate with parsley or scallion and serve.

One sliced umeboshi plum can be used instead of sauerkraut.

87. Broccoli, Carrot, Corn, and Shiitake Kanten

Serves 4

4 cups vegetable water
1 slice kombu, each 1"x 6"
3 sliced shiitake mushrooms (soak 10 minutes if dried and use the water)
2 tablespoons kuzu
1 cup cold water
1/2 cup brown rice vinegar
1 tablespoon tamari
1 teaspoon fresh ginger juice
2 tablespoons agar-agar flakes
Kernels from 1 cooked ear of corn
2 cups cooked broccoli heads, cut small
1 medium, cooked carrot, sliced in flowers

1. Add kombu and mushrooms to water. Bring to a boil. Simmer 20 minutes.

2. Remove kombu, slice into fine 1/4" squares and return to pot. Simmer 10 minutes.

3. Mix kuzu in water and stir into mixture.

4. Add rice vinegar, tamari, and ginger juice. Bring to a boil.

5. Add agar-agar flakes and stir well. Turn off heat.

6. Wet inside surface of a clean Pyrex dish or mold and pour in mixture.

7. Arrange corn, broccoli, and carrot flowers decoratively in the kanten and allow to cool, then refrigerate for an hour.

88. Broccoli with Roasted Pumpkin Seeds

Serves 2 to 4

2 tablespoons pumpkin seeds
4 cups broccoli florets (remove large stems and use for soups or stews)
1 1/2 cups water
1 tablespoon umeboshi vinegar

1. Place pumpkin seeds in iron skillet and roast over medium heat for 3 minutes.

2. Bring water to a boil. Add broccoli. Do not cover. Simmer for 5 minutes.

3. Strain off water and use it for making soup.

4. Sprinkle broccoli with seeds and umeboshi and serve. Lower stems can be boiled in the vegetable water for 10 minutes and used as a vegetable or for soup.

89. Carrageen Vegetable Aspic

Serves 4

3 cups water
1 cup soaked and washed carrageen
1 cup water
1/2 cup green peas
1 cup diced, peeled pumpkin
1/2 cup bean sprouts
1/2 cup sliced daikon
1 teaspoon grated lemon peel
1 tablespoon sauerkraut
Juice of half a lemon
1 tablespoon chopped parsley, to decorate

1. Bring water to a boil and add carrageen. Simmer for half an hour.
2. Meanwhile, in another pan, steam peas and pumpkin for 10 minutes (keep the steaming water).

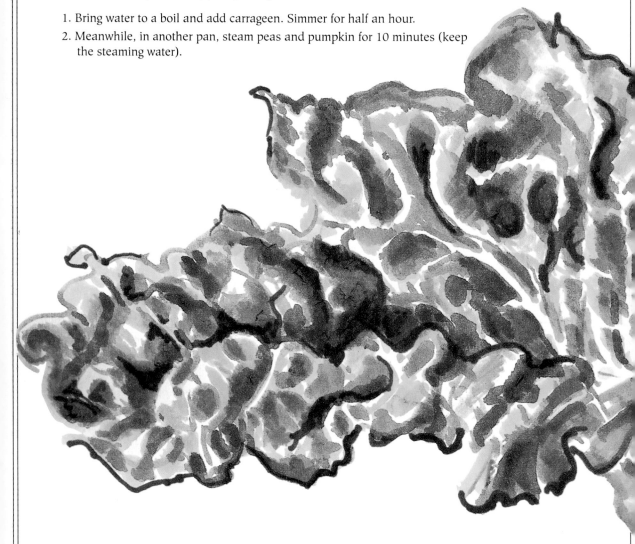

3. Place the vegetables in a flat dish and arrange bean sprouts, daikon, lemon peel, and sauerkraut over them.

4. Strain off water from carrageen (keep the carrageen and use for soups, aspics, etc.).

5. Mix hot carrageen water with 1/2 cup vegetable water and pour over the vegetables in dish. Let sit for 1/2 hour until cool. Refrigerate for 20 minutes.

6. Squeeze lemon juice over aspic, decorate with parsley and serve as salad with hot or cold rice or noodles.

90. Carrot, Apple, and Onion Salad with Raisins

Serves 4

A summer salad.

> 1 grated carrot
> 1 onion, finely diced
> 1 apple, diced
> 3/4 cup diced melon
> 1/2 cup diced tofu
> 1/2 cup apple juice
> 1 tablespoon umeboshi vinegar
> 1 teaspoon olive oil
> 1 teaspoon tamari
> 1/2 cup chopped parsley

1. Mix carrot, onion, apple, melon, and tofu.

2. Mix apple juice, vinegar, oils, and tamari.

3. Garnish with parsley and serve with cold brown rice.

91. Carrot, Dulse, and Celery Boiled Salad with Brown Rice Vinegar

Side dish for 4

> 1 cup dulse, soaked and cleaned
> 2 carrots, sliced in strips
> 3 stalks celery, sliced
> 2 cups boiling water
> 1 tablespoon brown rice vinegar
> 2 teaspoons roasted pine nuts

1. Slice soaked dulse.

2. Place dulse, carrots, and celery in pan.

3. Pour boiling water over vegetables and blanch for 30 seconds.

4. Remove vegetables (use water for soup).

5. Sprinkle with brown rice vinegar and roasted pine nuts. Serve.

92. Carrot and Scallion Salad

Side dish for 4

> 4 carrots, finely grated
> 5 scallions, finely chopped
> 1 tablespoon rice vinegar
> 1 tablespoon olive oil
> Pinch of salt

1. Mix carrots and scallions in a bowl.

2. Mix vinegar, oil, and salt in a separate bowl.

3. Pour dressing over vegetables and mix well. Let stand for 10 minutes in refrigerator.
Serve as a salad or decorate with Snow Pea and Ginger Salad (*see* Recipe 108).

93. Carrot and Turnip Cooked "Salad" in Umeboshi Vinegar

Side dish for 4

> 2 carrots, sliced
> 2 turnips, sliced
> 2 cups water
> 1/2 tablespoon umeboshi vinegar
> 1 teaspoon sesame salt

1. Boil carrots and turnips in water for 5 to 6 minutes, or until tender.

2. Strain off water (keep for soup).

3. Sprinkle with umeboshi vinegar and sesame salt.

94. Boiled Cauliflower and Kuzu Salad

Side dish for 4

>1 small cauliflower head
>1 cup water
>2 tablespoons umeboshi vinegar
>2 teaspoons kuzu
>1 cup cold water

1. Break up the cauliflower into small florets.
2. Bring water to a boil and place heads in it. Simmer for 3 minutes, until tender. Use this water for sauce.
3. Place the cooked cauliflower in dish to cool.
4. Using cauliflower water, add umeboshi vinegar and heat.
5. Dissolve kuzu in 1 cup cold water and add to the umeboshi water. Just bring to a boil, stirring all the time, and remove from heat.
6. Pour sauce over the cauliflower florets.

95. Cauliflower in Umeboshi Vinegar

Side dish for 4

>3 cups cauliflower florets
>1 cup salted water
>1/4 cup umeboshi vinegar
>1/4 cup water

1. Break the cauliflower into florets rather than cut them.
2. Place florets in the boiling salted water for about 2 minutes (until tender).
3. Take out and allow to cool (keep water for soup stock).
4. Mix the umeboshi vinegar with an equal amount of water, place the cauliflower florets in the mixture and let stand for 20 to 30 minutes. Stir.
5. Take cauliflower out of the vinegar solution and serve.

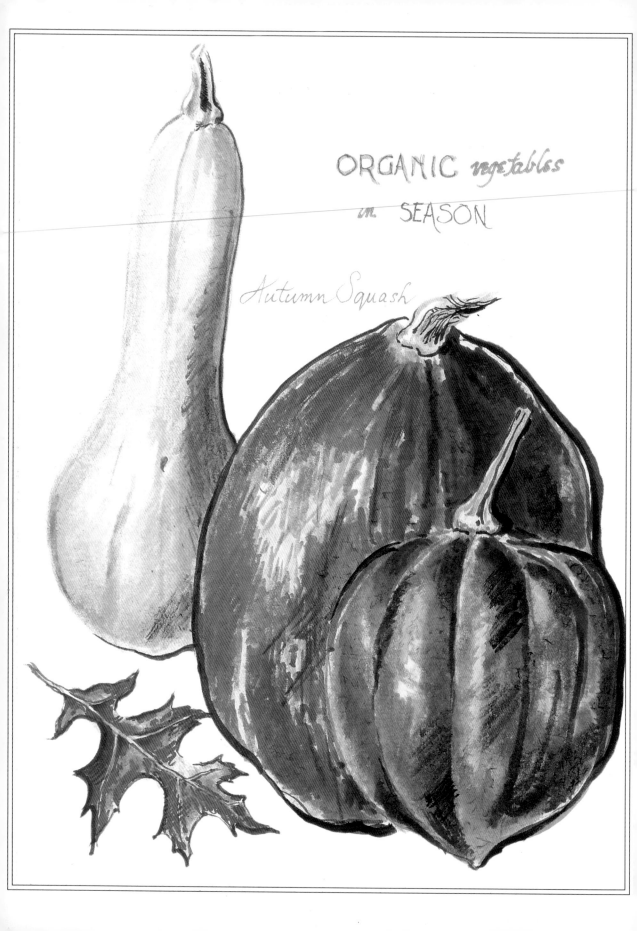

ORGANIC vegetables in SEASON

Autumn Squash

96. Cauliflower, Yellow Squash, and Leeks with Chickpeas

Serves 4

    1 cup chickpeas
    3 cups soaking water
    1/2 cup sliced dulse
    4 cups water
    1 tablespoon olive oil
    1 cup roll cut parsnip
    1 cup chopped leek
    1 clove garlic, chopped
    1" ginger, grated fine
    3 cups cauliflower florets
    1 tablespoon fresh, chopped dill
    1 teaspoon fresh tarragon, chopped fine
    1 small, yellow summer squash, sliced in rounds
    3 sliced leaves spinach (or kale)
    1 tablespoon tamari
    1/2 cup chopped, roasted walnuts

1. Soak chickpeas overnight. Discard water, replace with 4 cups fresh, and cook with dulse for 3 hours (*see* INGREDIENTS—Legumes).
2. Place oil in a pan and heat gently. Add parsnip, leek, garlic, and ginger. Sauté, stirring well, for 10 minutes.
3. Add cauliflower, dill, and tarragon and sauté, covered for 5 minutes.
4. Add squash and spinach (or kale), replace lid and simmer for 10 minutes.
5. Stir in tamari, sprinkle on walnuts, and serve on a bed of brown rice or millet.

97. Chinese Hand-Pressed Cabbage Salad

Side dish for 4

This salad can be made quickly.

    1/4 Chinese cabbage
    1 teaspoon salt
    2 tablespoons umeboshi vinegar
    1 sprig parsley, chopped

1. Slice the cabbage lengthwise, then very finely across.
2. Sprinkle with the salt and press by hand, squeezing out water.
3. When it is well pressed, strain off the cabbage water and rinse cabbage with fresh, running water.
4. Place in bowl and mix in umeboshi vinegar.
5. Decorate with chopped parsley and serve.

98. Chinese Pressed Cabbage Salad

Side dish for 4

You will need a salad press for this recipe.

> 1/2 Chinese cabbage, finely sliced
> 2 teaspoons tamari
> 2 teaspoons juice of grated ginger

1. Press cabbage by hand into press.
2. Pour tamari and ginger juice over cabbage in press.
3. Leave pressed for 1 hour. (The pressure also helps to "yangize" the cabbage.)
4. Drain off water, rinse if preferred and serve.

99. Daikon and Umeboshi Vinegar

Side dish for 4

> 2 cups grated daikon
> 2 teaspoons umeboshi vinegar

1. Sprinkle the umeboshi vinegar over the grated daikon. It will turn a delicate pink color.
2. Makes a clean-tasting side dish, to be served with a grain meal or with meat.

100. Hijiki-Shiitake Side Dish

Serves 4 to 6

> 1 cup hijiki
> 3 cups water
> 1 medium onion, sliced
> 1 carrot, matchstick sliced
> 1 tablespoon toasted sesame oil
> 4 shiitake mushrooms, sliced. (If dried soak in 2 cups water for 10 minutes and remove stalk ends. Save soaking water.)
> 1 cup apple juice
> 2 teaspoons tamari
> 1 teaspoon fresh, ginger juice
> Parsley, to garnish

1. Soak hijiki for 10 minutes in 1 cup water. Strain off water and set aside.
2. Sauté onion and carrot in sesame oil until onion is transparent (5 minutes).
3. Add hijiki, shiitake, and soaking water plus 1 cup apple juice to cover vegetables. Bring to a boil, cover, and simmer gently for 45 minutes.
4. Stir in tamari and ginger juice. Simmer another 15 minutes to evaporate most of the liquid.
5. Garnish with parsley and serve hot as a side dish or chilled over a bed of lettuce.

101. Hijiki with Onion, Carrots, and Nuts

Serves 4 to 6

> 1 cup hijiki
> 4 cups water
> 1 tablespoon sunflower oil
> 1 onion, sliced
> 1 grated carrot or 1 cup diced pumpkin (peeled)
> 1/2 cup cashew nuts
> 1 tablespoon pine nuts
> 2 teaspoons miso
> 1/2 cup boiling water

1. Soak hijiki in 2 cups water, until soft (10 minutes).

2. Strain off water and keep it.

3. Place oil in a deep pan, heat gently, and put in onion; stir until golden brown. Add the hijiki and stir well for 5 minutes.

4. Add the hijiki soaking water and the 2 extra cups of water and bring to a boil. Simmer for 40 minutes, or until most of the water has boiled away.

5. Add the grated carrot or pumpkin, water, and nuts. Mix gently. Let simmer for 10 minutes, or until carrot or pumpkin is soft.

6. Mix miso well in 1/2 cup water and add to the hijiki, stirring well.

7. Serve as a side dish or use as a stuffing for cabbage.

102. Hijiki and Ginger

Serves 4 to 6

> 1 cup hijiki
> 4 cups water
> 1 teaspoon safflower oil
> 2 tablespoons tamari
> 1 tablespoon fresh, grated ginger
> 1/2 cup goat yogurt (optional)

1. Rinse hijiki; then soak in 2 cups water for 10 minutes.

2. Stain off and keep the water.

3. Sauté hijiki in the oil for 10 minutes.

4. Add tamari, ginger, and the straining water and bring to a boil; turn down heat and simmer for 40 minutes, or until water has evaporated.

5. Sprinkle each serving with parsley and a squeeze of lemon juice. Decorate with a teaspoon of goat yogurt (optional).

If served cold, sautéed (or raw) grated carrot may be added for variety.

103. Kale and Mushrooms Boiled

Serves 4

> 6 kale leaves
> 1 cup water
> 6 shiitake mushrooms, dried or fresh
> 2 teaspoons tamari
> 1/2 cup water
> 1 tablespoon freshly roasted sesame seeds

1. Steam or boil the kale leaves, whole, for 3 to 4 minutes in water until tender. Then slice fine. (Save the water for soup.)

2. If dried shiitake mushrooms are used, soak them for 10 minutes. Place mushrooms in 1/2 cup water and tamari. Allow to simmer without cover for 15 minutes. Slice. Remove shiitake stems if tough.

3. Mix sliced kale with mushrooms and sesame seeds and serve.

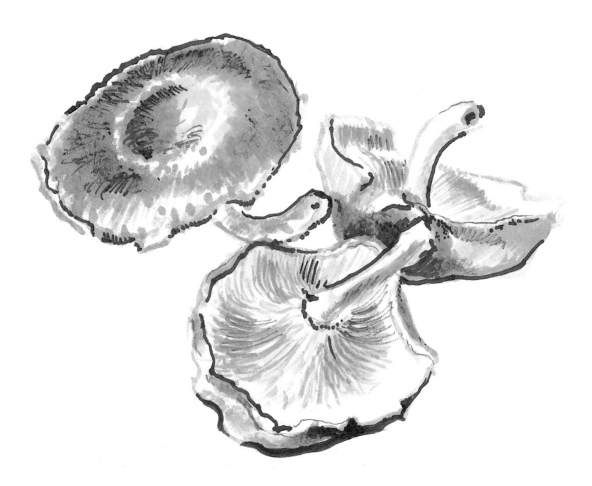

104. Kale Water-Sautéed

Serves 4

Vegetables are delicious if sautéed vigorously for a couple of minutes in a *little* boiling water.

> 12 leaves curly kale, sliced
> 1/2 cup water
> Pinch of salt
> 1 tablespoon roasted pumpkin seeds

1. Bring salted water to a boil and keep heat at medium.
2. Add kale and stir. Keep it moving for 3 minutes, or until the color suddenly becomes intensely green. It should then be tender.
3. Sprinkle with pumpkin seeds and serve immediately.

105. Kampyo-Kale Bundles

Serves 4

Kampyo is made from dried strips of gourd skin. It looks very much like a grain or pasta but is, in fact, a vegetable.

> 8 ounces gourd strips (kampyo)
> 3 cups boiling water
> 1 tablespoon tamari
> 8 ounces kale leaves, with stem
> Pinch of salt
> 2 cups water

1. Soak kampyo for 10 minutes.
2. Boil the gourd strips gently for 45 minutes in water and tamari.
3. Place kale leaves in salted boiling water for 3 to 4 minutes. Remove (keep water for soup stock).
4. Tie the leaves by the stems with the gourd strips in a tidy bow.
5. Serve the bundles with a main grain dish and vegetables.

106. Kombu and Carrots

Serves 4 to 6

> 1 1/2 cups water
> 1/2 cup soaked kombu, cut into 1/4" squares
> 2 teaspoons tamari
> 2 carrots
> 2 teaspoons safflower oil

1. Bring water to a boil, add kombu, and simmer over low heat for 20 minutes. Add more water if necessary.
2. Add tamari and boil another 10 minutes, or until most of the liquid has evaporated.
3. Meanwhile slice carrots into rounds and sauté in 1 teaspoon oil for 5 minutes. Add kombu and sauté with carrots until they are soft.

Wakame can be used instead of kombu. It will take less time to cook—10 minutes instead of 30.

107. Lentil Pâté

Serves 4

Great for a party!

>3 cups water
>1 strip kombu
>2 cups lentils
>1 bay leaf
>2 1/2 cups sourdough bread (see Recipe 73)
>2 cups water
>2 large onions, sliced
>2 tablespoons olive oil
>3/4 cup fresh, chopped parsley
>1 teaspoon fresh sage (1/2 teaspoon dried)
>2 teaspoons fresh thyme (1 teaspoon dried)
>1/4 cup tahini
>1 tablespoon genmai miso

1. Preheat oven to 350°F/180°C.
2. Bring water and kombu to a boil, add lentils and bay leaf and simmer for 40 minutes, or until lentils are soft.
3. Remove bay leaf and blend.
4. Soak bread for 20 minutes in water. Drain off and keep water and blend the bread and lentils.
5. Sauté onions for 5 minutes in the olive oil
6. Add parsley and herbs. Sauté 5 minutes.
7. Meanwhile mix tahini and miso with 1/2 cup of the bread water.
8. Mix the onions, herbs, tahini and miso with the bread and lentils and stir well.
9. Place in an oiled pan and bake for 40 minutes in preheated oven.

108. Snow Pea and Ginger Salad

Serves 4

>1 tablespoon toasted sesame oil
>1/2 pound snow peas
>1 tablespoon fresh ginger juice
>1 teaspoon tamari

1. Gently heat oil in a pan.
2. Sauté snow peas for 5 minutes.
3. Add ginger juice. Stir for 2 minutes.
4. Turn off heat. Add 1 teaspoon tamari.
5. Serve as a salad or use to decorate other vegetable salads (*see* Recipe 92).

109. Mustard Greens with Pumpkin Seed Salad

Serves 4

> 3 cups sliced mustard greens
> 1 cup water
> 1/2 cup toasted pumpkin seeds
> 3 tablespoons sweet rice vinegar

1. Place water in a pot and the greens in a steamer. Cover and steam vegetables for 10 to 15 minutes.
2. Place cooked greens in a bowl. Save the water for soup.
3. Sprinkle the pumpkin seeds over greens and garnish with the rice vinegar. Serve hot or cold.

110. Nori "Black Butter" and Mushrooms on Toast

Serves 2 to 3

Use as a spread. Good with hummus on bannock or bread.

> 2 sheets nori
> 1 teaspoon sesame oil
> 1 small onion, sliced
> 2 medium mushrooms, sliced (optional)
> 1 cup water
> 1 teaspoon kuzu
> 1 tablespoon tamari
> 2 to 3 slices whole wheat bread, toasted
> 2 to 3 slices of lemon
> Sprig of parsley

1. Break up the nori sheets into small pieces.
2. Heat oil in pan, place onion and mushrooms in and sauté gently.
3. Add nori and stir for a minute.
4. Pour in 1/2 cup water and stir well. Boil for 5 minutes.
5. Mix kuzu in 1/2 cup water. Add kuzu and tamari to the nori. Stir. Bring almost to a boil.
6. Serve on slices of whole wheat toast with a slice of lemon and a sprinkling of tamari. Garnish with parsley.

III. Pancakes with Béchamel Vegetable Sauce

Serves 4

> 1 cup chopped white cabbage
> 1 small carrot, finely diced
> 1/2 cup chopped scallions
> 1/2 cup bean sprouts
> 1 cup water
> 1 cup soy milk
> 1 tablespoon kuzu
> Pinch of salt
> 1 tablespoon rice vinegar
> 1/2 cup chopped parsley

1. Boil cabbage, carrot, scallions, and bean sprouts gently in water for 5 minutes.

2. Mix kuzu in soy milk with salt and rice vinegar and add to the vegetables to thicken. Bring to a boil, stirring until sauce thickens. Turn off heat.

3. Make pancakes (*see* Recipe 80). Place one pancake on a plate and cover with sauce. Add next pancake on top of this, cover with sauce, and repeat until last pancake is used. Garnish with any remaining sauce, decorate with parsley, and serve. Slice as you would a cake.

II2. Parsnips and Onion Baked with Parsley and Mochi Sauce

Side dish for 4

> 2 medium parsnips, sliced diagonally
> 1 large onion, sliced
> 2 teaspoons sesame oil
> Pinch of salt
> 1/2 cup grated mochi
> 1 cup water
> 1 teaspoon tahini
> 2 teaspoons tamari
> 1 tablespoon rice vinegar
> 2 tablespoons chopped parsley

1. Preheat oven to 350°F/180°C.

2. Gently sauté onion and parsnips in oil for 5 minutes. Ensure that they are lightly and evenly covered and slightly cooked.

3. Sprinkle on salt and place in a shallow dish in a preheated oven for 1/2 hour.

4. Make sauce by adding mochi to 1 cup boiling water over heat.

5. Add tahini and tamari to the mixture, stirring well.

6. Simmer and stir in rice vinegar and parsley.

7. Cover parsnips and onion with the sauce and serve as a side dish.

113. Parsley in Tempura Batter

Garnish for 4 to 6

> 6 sprigs fresh parsley
> 2 tablespoons whole wheat pastry flour
> 1 tablespoon yellow cornmeal
> Pinch of salt
> 1 tablespoon kuzu in 1 cup cold water
> 1 1/2 cups cold water
> 1/2 cup sesame oil

1. Wash parsley. Dry it in a cloth.

2. Mix whole wheat flour, cornmeal, and salt.

3. Dissolve kuzu in cup of cold water.

4. Add kuzu and water and extra water to flour to make batter. Let stand in a cool place for an hour before using.

5. Dip parsley into batter and fry quickly in hot oil. Oil should not be too hot. (*See* INGREDI-ENTS—Tempura.)

Other vegetables can also be cooked in this way. Serve as a garnish with grains or soup.

114. Pickled Dill Cucumber

Pickling is, of course, an ancient method of preserving food naturally. It also helps digestion, and there are many recipes for preparing pickles. Sea salt, pressure, and time yangize the food. Salted pickles can be purchased in most natural food stores, but here is a recipe for making them.

Makes 2 or 3 1-pint jars

> 4 cups water to cover
> 1/3 cup sea salt
> 2 pounds small pickling cucumbers
> 1 large onion, sliced
> 2 sprigs fresh or dry dill

1. Gently boil salt and water for 2 minutes, until salt dissolves. Allow to cool.

2. Wash cucumbers and place in pickling jars with onion and dill. Pour cooled salt water over them to cover.

3. Leave uncovered in a dark, cool place for 3 to 4 days.

4. Place in jars and refrigerate—they will keep for a month or so.

115. Pickled Sauerkraut

> 1 1/2 pound head of cabbage (4 cups grated)
> 1 tablespoon sea salt

1. Wash cabbage well. Dry and slice very thin.

2. Place in a wooden keg or china crock and sprinkle with salt.

3. Cover with a wooden dish or plate, slightly smaller than the container opening, so that when a weight is placed on it there is pressure on the cabbage. Cover with cheesecloth and leave in a cool, dark place.

4. After 10 hours or so, water should cover the cabbage. If not, increase weight.

5. Check daily. If mold forms, remove it—it is not harmful but can affect the flavor.

6. After two weeks, rinse the cabbage in cold water. It is now ready for use.

116. Potato and Leek Salad

Serves 4

Just for a change!

> 1 pound small, organic red potatoes
> 2 cups water
> Pinch of salt
> 2 leek tops, finely sliced
> Juice of 1/2 lemon
> 1 tablespoon olive oil

1. Boil potatoes in water and salt for 20 minutes, or until tender.

2. Cut potatoes in half. Allow to cool.

3. Add the very finely sliced leek tops.

4. Toss the vegetables in olive oil and lemon juice and serve.

117. Pressed Carrot, Daikon, and Cucumber Salad

Serves 4

A refreshing side dish or eat with bannocks and hummus.

> 1 medium carrot
> 1 4"to 5" cucumber
> 6 radishes or a 3" piece of daikon
> 1 teaspoon umeboshi vinegar or 1 pinch sea salt

1. Wash and scrub vegetables well.

2. Grate vegetables into bowl or deep plate and sprinkle with umeboshi or salt.

3. Place a slightly smaller bowl or plate into the container and stand a heavy weight on top.

4. Press salad for at least 45 minutes.

5. Strain off juice, stir ingredients, and rinse if preferred. Serve.

This salad can be used as the chief ingredient of Brown Rice Summer Salad (*see* Recipe 38).

118. Radishes, Dulse, and Daikon Salad

Serves 4

>6 radishes, finely sliced
>1 cup finely sliced daikon
>2 tablespoons umeboshi vinegar
>1 cup boiling water
>1 cup dulse (washed)
>1/2 cup boiling water

1. Blanch radishes and daikon in boiling water. Strain (keep water for soups).
2. Sprinkle with umeboshi vinegar.
3. Pour boiling water over dulse. Stir and leave for a minute. Strain dulse (keep water for soup). Add dulse to radishes and daikon and mix together.
4. Serve as a side salad.

119. Radish Flowers and Umeboshi Kanten

>12 radishes
>1 cup boiling water
>3 cups vegetable water or 3 cups water with a pinch of kombu powder
>2 tablespoons umeboshi vinegar
>2 teaspoons agar-agar flakes
>1 tablespoon tamari

1. Slice radishes into flowers. Cut bottom across (so they stand straight).
2. Blanch in boiling water. Flowers will then open up. Remove and stand in umeboshi vinegar (keep water).
3. Heat vegetable water or water and kombu with blanching water, tamari, and umeboshi vinegar. Sprinkle agar-agar flakes over and stir well. Turn off heat just before boiling.
4. Rinse shallow Pyrex dish in cold water and pour the vegetable water and agar-agar into it. It should be deep enough to cover the radishes.
5. When it has partly set, push radishes in to form a pattern. Allow to cool and set.
6. Turn out of the dish, slice to serve.

120. Red Cabbage, Apple, and Umeboshi

Serves 4

>1 tablespoon corn oil
>1 small, red cabbage, sliced fine
>2 cups apple juice
>2 tablespoons umeboshi vinegar
>1 apple, diced
>3/4 cup sultanas or raisins

1. Heat oil in a skillet and add cabbage. Stir gently over medium-low heat for 2 minutes.
2. Add apple juice, umeboshi vinegar, apple, and sultanas or raisins. Bring to a boil. Simmer slowly over low heat for 45 minutes.
3. Stir and serve. The umeboshi vinegar keeps the cabbage a bright red color.

121. Sauerkraut, Avocado, Aduki, and Ulva Kanten Salad

Side dish for 4

> 1 cup sauerkraut (*see* Recipe 115)
> 1 umeboshi plum, chopped fine
> 1/2 avocado, sliced
> 2 tablespoons cooked aduki beans
> 1/2 cup soaked ulva (sea lettuce)
> 2 teaspoons agar-agar flakes
> 1 cup water (vegetable water preferred)
> 1 tablespoon tamari
> 1/2 cup chopped parsley or sliced scallions, to garnish

1. Mix sauerkraut and umeboshi. Place in wet salad bowl.
2. Spread slices of avocado over sauerkraut.
3. Sprinkle aduki beans around this and place ulva on top.
4. Mix agar-agar flakes in hot water, stir, and bring gently to boiling point. Turn off heat and add tamari.
5. Allow agar-agar water to cool slightly and pour over the vegetables. Let set 10 to 15 minutes. Refrigerate for 20 minutes.
6. Turn out kanten onto plate and garnish with parsley or sliced scallions.

122. Sauerkraut and Radish Kanten

Side dish for 4

> 2 cups boiling water
> 1 heaping teaspoon agar-agar
> 2 tablespoons sauerkraut
> 6 or 8 large red radishes, sliced
> 1 umeboshi plum, chopped

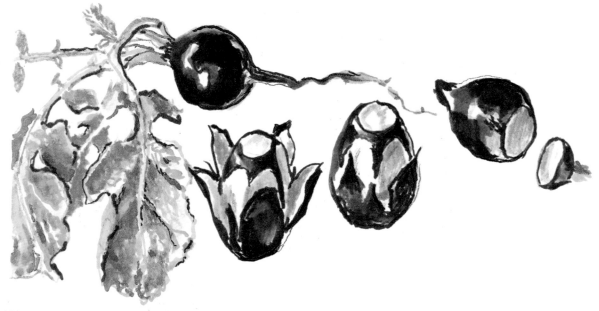

1 sprig parsley
Chopped parsley, to garnish

1. Let water simmer gently over low heat. Add agar-agar. Stir until dissolved.
2. Turn off heat. Add sauerkraut, sliced radishes, and umeboshi. Stir well.
3. Wet the inside of a shallow earthenware or Pyrex dish with cold water to prevent the kanten from sticking when it sets. Pour in the mixture.
4. Leave to set for 10 to 20 minutes at room temperature. Refrigerate for 20 minutes.
5. Turn out onto a shallow plate, decorate with parsley, and serve as a side dish.

123. Sauerkraut on Toast

Serves 4

4 slices bread
1 teaspoon olive oil
1 tablespoon tahini spread
1 cup sauerkraut

1. Fry bread lightly in oil on both sides and then spread with tahini. Heat under broiler (grill) for 1 minute.
2. Place sauerkraut in pan and simmer for 2 minutes. Serve spread on the bread.

124. Sushi Nori Roll with Tempeh, Ginger, Carrot, and Scallion

Serves 4 to 6

4 slices cooked tempeh each 1/4" wide by 6" long
1 carrot, sliced lengthwise into 1/4" strips
1/2 cup water
1/2 tablespoon dark sesame oil
2 tablespoons ginger juice

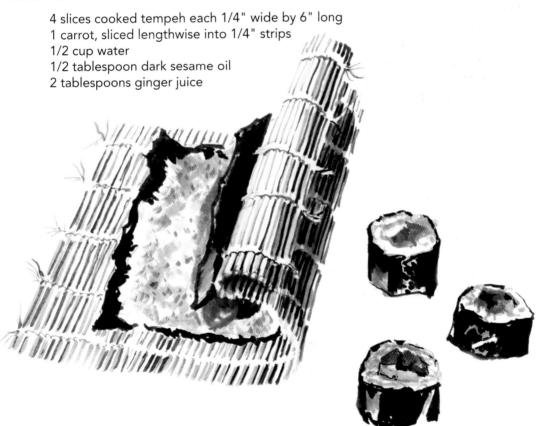

3 cups soft, cooked brown rice
2 tablespoons rice vinegar
2 tablespoons lemon juice
4 sheets nori
1 scallion sliced fine into 6" lengths

1. Prepare tempeh in pan, as for recipe 132.

2. Bring the carrot to a boil in 1/2 cup water and simmer gently in covered pan until soft (15 minutes) and water has evaporated. Add dark sesame oil and ginger juice and sauté another 5 minutes.

3. Mix rice vinegar and lemon juice into the rice.

4. Toast sheets of nori gently over a low flame until a deep green color and crisp.

5. Place a sheet of nori on your sushi mat. The soft rice should be evenly spread about 1/2" from the edge of the sheet and 1" from the top and bottom. You are making four rolls, so use a quarter quantity of each ingredient.

6. Wet your hands and make a groove across the rice, 1 1/2" from the bottom, into which you can layer the tempeh and ginger, carrot and scallion.

7. Roll the sushi in a mat as though making a long cigarette. Keep it firm, even, and smooth.

8. Use a very sharp knife to slice each roll across into bite-sized pieces (about 3/4" wide).

Serve with a dip of tamari with a touch of wasabi horseradish, mixing the wasabi powder with a few drops of water. (*See also* INGREDIENTS—Sushi.)

125. Sweet Boiled Carrots

Serves 2 to 4

One of the best ways to cook carrots

3 cups sliced carrots
Water to almost cover
Parsley or peas, to garnish

1. Place carrots in enough water to almost cover them. Leave lid off pot.

2. Bring to a boil and cook gently for 20 minutes, or until the water has evaporated. Do not stir, but shake the pot to stop sticking if necessary.

3. Decorate with parsley or peas and serve.

126. Ulva, Dulse, and Orange Salad

Serves 4

1 cup washed ulva and dulse
1 cup boiling water
1 orange, peeled
3/4 cup apple juice
1 umeboshi plum, pitted and sliced
1 teaspoon white shiro miso
3 cups cooked and strained soba or udon noodles (*see* INGREDIENTS—Noodles)
3/4 cup watercress

1. Wash ulva and dulse thoroughly and slice into pieces. Pour a cup of boiling water over them. Let stand for a minute. Strain off water and keep for soups.

2. Remove most of the outside pith from the orange and slice finely.

3. Mix apple juice and umeboshi plum with miso for dressing salad.

4. Chop cooked noodles into 2 to 3" lengths and place in bowl. Cover with ulva, dulse, orange, and dressing. Mix together until evenly coated with dressing.

5. Garnish with watercress. This can stand for an hour before serving.

127. Umeboshi-Kuzu Vegetables

Serves 2

>   6 fresh mushrooms, sliced
>   1 small zucchini, sliced
>   8 small, young spinach leaves
>   1 1/2 cups water
>   2 teaspoons kuzu
>   1/2 cup cold water
>   1 umeboshi plum, sliced
>   1/2 teaspoon gomasio (*see* INGREDIENTS—Gomasio)

1. Place vegetables in a steamer.

2. Bring water to a boil and steam vegetables for 5 minutes, until tender. Remove from pan.

3. Mix kuzu in 1/2 cup cold water. Add with umeboshi slices to the vegetable water. Bring gently to boiling point, stirring until liquid is clear. Add vegetables, sprinkle with gomasio, and serve with boiled rice or rice croquettes.

128. Watercress, Orange, and Scallion Salad

Side dish for 4

>   3 cups watercress
>   1 scallion, sliced fine (use all of it)
>   1/2 cup apple juice
>   1 teaspoon sesame oil
>   1 teaspoon tamari
>   1 umeboshi plum, sliced
>   1 orange, peeled

1. Wash watercress thoroughly and drain. Place in salad bowl.

2. Add scallion to watercress.

3. Mix apple juice, oil, tamari, and umeboshi plum for dressing salad.

4. Remove skin and most of the outside white pith from the orange and slice finely.

5. Pour dressing over the salad and stir. Decorate with the oranges and serve.

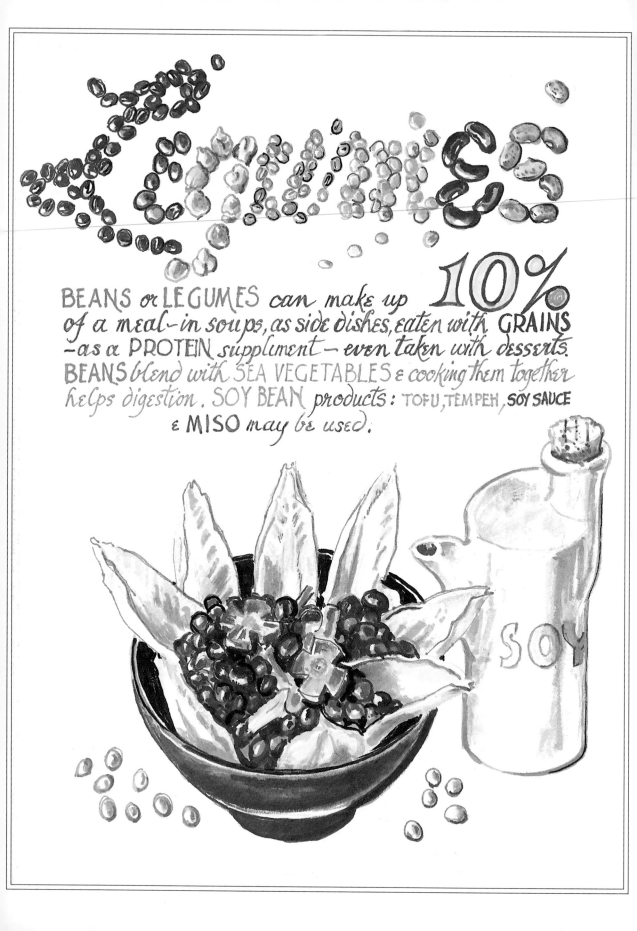

Legumes

BEANS or LEGUMES can make up **10%** of a meal – in soups, as side dishes, eaten with GRAINS – as a PROTEIN supplement – even taken with desserts. BEANS blend with SEA VEGETABLES & cooking them together helps digestion. SOY BEAN products: TOFU, TEMPEH, **SOY SAUCE** & MISO may be used.

SOY

Legumes

129. Aduki and Pumpkin

Side dish for 4 to 6

> 1 cup aduki beans
> 3/4 cup soaked and chopped wakame or 2 strips kombu, 6" x 2"
> 4 cups water
> 2 cups diced 1" pumpkin squares
> 1 onion, sliced
> 1/4 cup tamari
> Chopped parsley, to garnish

1. Wash aduki and soak for 1 or 2 hours. Discard water.
2. Wipe wakame strips (or kombu) with a damp cloth to remove excess salt as this will harden beans when cooking.
3. Place beans and wakame or kombu in pan, cover with fresh water and bring to a boil. Lower heat and simmer for 45 minutes.
4. Place onion and pumpkin on top and cook another 20 minutes.
5. Add tamari and turn up heat to boil off excess water.
6. Mix ingredients, garnish with parsley, and serve.

130. Aduki Pizza

Serves 4 to 6

> 1 cup aduki beans soaked in 3 cups water
> 1 slice kombu, 6"x 2"
> 4 cups water
> 1 teaspoon caraway seeds
> 1 onion, sliced
> 1 parsnip, diced
> 2 tablespoons tamari
> 6 olives
> 2 rings sweet red pepper
> 1 cup mochi-umeboshi sauce

1. Preheat oven to 350°F/180°C.
2. Soak aduki beans for 2 hours. Discard water.
3. Wipe excess salt from the kombu strip with a damp cloth.
4. Bring fresh water to a boil with aduki, kombu, and caraway seeds. Cover and simmer for 45 minutes.
5. Place onion and parsnip on top of aduki, cover, and continue to simmer for another 20 minutes. Add tamari. Boil off excess water.
6. Beans and parsnip should be soft enough to mash to make topping for pizza.
7. Spread aduki mixture on precooked pastry (*see* Recipe 79), cover with Mochi-Umeboshi Sauce (*see* Recipe 147) or Béchamel Sauce (*see* Recipe 137) and decorate with olives and pieces of red pepper.
8. Bake in preheated oven for 15 minutes.

This mixture could also be used on noodles or spaghetti.

131. Aduki, Rice, and Sweet Corn Croquettes

Serves 4 to 6

>1 cup water
>1 small onion, finely chopped
>1 small carrot, finely diced
>2 teaspoons tamari
>2 cups soft, cooked brown rice (*see* INGREDIENTS—Grains)
>1/2 cup sweet corn kernels
>1 cup soft, cooked aduki (or black) beans (*see* INGREDIENTS—Legumes)
>2 cups whole wheat bread crumbs
>1 tablespoon sesame or corn oil

1. Bring water to a boil. Add onion and carrot. Simmer for 10 minutes, or until vegetables are soft. Add tamari.
2. Mix rice, corn, and beans together. Add vegetables and enough of the water to make mixture stick together. Allow to cool.
3. Wet your hands and roll mixture into croquettes (4 or 6).
4. Roll croquettes in bread crumbs.
5. Brush skillet with oil and heat gently. Sauté croquettes until brown.
6. Serve with Mochi-Umeboshi Sauce (*see* Recipe 147) and garnish with parsley.

132. Tempeh, Ginger, and Tamari Slices

Serves 4 to 6

>4 ounces tempeh
>1 strip kombu in 1" squares
>2 tablespoons tamari
>1 tablespoon grated ginger
>2 cups apple juice

1. Slice tempeh into strips 3" x 1".
2. Place in pan with kombu, tamari, ginger, and apple juice.
3. Bring to a boil, lower heat, cover, and simmer for 40 minutes, or until most of the liquid has evaporated.
4. Use this tempeh for stews, sandwiches, or in Sushi rolls (*see* Recipe 124).

Can also be rolled in sesame or caraway seeds and shallow-fried in 1 teaspoon of sesame oil. Drain and serve with a natural mustard and grated daikon.

133. Tempeh and Mochi Layered Stew

Serves 4 to 6

>4 slices cooked tempeh in 1"x 2" strips
>6 slices mochi
>1 tablespoon safflower oil

Pinch of salt
1 tablespoon tamari
3/4 cup sliced burdock root (soaked)
1 cup water
1 cup sliced rutabaga
1/4 teaspoon kombu powder
1/2 Chinese cabbage, sliced
1 cup bean sprouts
1 cup watercress (washed)

1. Prepare tempeh as for Recipe 132.

2. Gently sauté mochi in the oil with salt until pieces burst and are golden brown (about 10 minutes). Sprinkle with tamari.

3. After soaking burdock root for 10 minutes, discard water and place slices in a pan with a cup of water, sprinkle on kombu powder, bring to a boil and simmer, uncovered, for 5 minutes.

4. Add tempeh, rutabaga, cabbage, bean sprouts, and watercress. Cover and simmer for 5 minutes.

6. Add mochi and serve with grains.

134. Tempeh with Tahini and Miso Cream Sauce

Serves 4

1 tablespoon light tahini
1 teaspoon kuzu in 1 cup cold water
1 tablespoon light shiro miso in 1/2 cup hot water
8 ounces tempeh, prepared as in Recipe 132 and sliced into 1/2" squares

1. Heat tahini in pan and stir until it begins to bubble.

2. Having mixed miso in hot water and kuzu in cold water, add to the tahini. Stir until sauce thickens. It should be smooth—add water if necessary.

3. Add tempeh and stir.

4. Serve over brown rice or grains with a side dish of hot vegetables or salad.

135. Tofu on Sautéed Onion

Side dish for 4

8 slices of tofu, 2" squares 1/4" thick
1 tablespoon safflower oil
2 medium onions, sliced
1/2 cup water
1 teaspoon tamari
2 teaspoons fresh ginger juice

1. Heat skillet brushed with oil and gently sauté tofu until golden brown.

2. In another pan sauté onions in rest of oil for 3 minutes or until golden brown.

3. Add water, tamari, and ginger.

4. Serve tofu on the bed of onions.

Fried tofu can also be used in soups, stews, or on other vegetables.

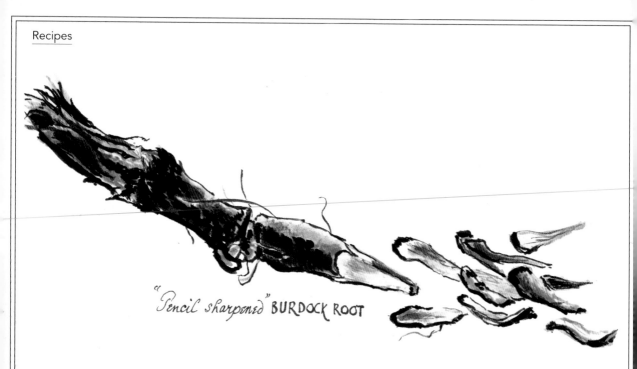

"Pencil sharpened" BURDOCK ROOT

136. Tofu Sticks Sautéed with Burdock and Vegetables

Serves 2 to 4

>1 tablespoon sesame oil
>8 slices of tofu, 1/2" x 1"
>1/2 cup finely pencil-sliced fresh burdock root
>1 teaspoon toasted sesame oil
>1 onion, sliced
>1 small carrot, sliced
>1 strip sweet red pepper, chopped
>1 cup water
>1 teaspoon kuzu
>1/2 cup water

1. Brush skillet with oil and place in tofu slices. Sauté and turn gently over medium-low heat until golden brown.

2. Soak burdock root for 10 minutes in a little water. Discard water.

3. Sauté burdock root in rest of oil for 10 minutes. Add onion, carrot, and pepper. Stir-fry for 10 minutes. Pour in 1 cup water. Simmer for 15 minutes.

4. Dissolve kuzu in water and add to vegetables. Sauce should not be too thick; add more water if necessary.

5. Serve vegetables with tofu and brown rice.

Sauces, Spreads, and Dips

137. Béchamel Sauce

      1 1/2 tablespoons whole wheat flour
      1 cup water
      1 cup rice or oat milk
      1 tablespoon umeboshi vinegar or 1 tablespoon fresh ginger juice or 1 tablespoon fresh lemon juice
      1 tablespoon tamari
      2 teaspoons kuzu
      1/2 cup water

1. Mix flour in the cold water and heat gently, stirring well.
2. Add half the milk and the umeboshi vinegar (or ginger juice or lemon juice) with tamari. Bring to a boil. The flour should thicken slightly. Add rest of the milk.
3. Mix the kuzu in cold water and pour into the mixture, stirring well, until it thickens into a smooth sauce.
4. Serve over vegetables, rice, noodles, or fish.

The above sauce can be used as a base for:

Cheese Sauce—Add 1 tablespoon of grated provolone or goat cheese with tahini umeboshi vinegar.

Parsley Sauce—Add 2 tablespoons of chopped parsley with ginger juice.

Onion Sauce—Add a small chopped onion with umeboshi vinegar.

Mushroom Sauce—Add 1 small chopped onion and 1 cup sliced mushrooms with ginger juice.

Lemon Sauce—Add 1 teaspoon grated lemon rind with lemon juice.

138. Black Bean and Chickpea Pâté

Serves 4 to 6

      1/2 cup cooked chickpeas with kombu
      1/2 cup black turtle beans
      1 strip kombu, 3"x 1"
      4 cups water
      1 clove garlic, chopped
      2 tablespoons soy sauce
      1 teaspoon caraway seeds
      1/4 green pepper, sliced
      1/2 cup chopped parsley

1. Soak chickpeas overnight. Soak turtle beans for 1 hour. Drain and discard water.
2. Add kombu to 4 cups fresh water and bring to a boil. Add beans and chickpeas.
3. Boil for 3 hours, or until chickpeas are soft.
4. Add garlic, soy sauce, and caraway seeds. Blend. Decorate with parsley and green pepper and serve with whole wheat crackers or bread.

139. Cabbage and Caraway-Tofu Sauce

Serves 6

>1/2 small, hard white cabbage
>1/2 cup water
>1 teaspoon caraway seeds
>1 cup tofu pieces
>2 umeboshi plums, seeded
>2 teaspoons kuzu in 1/2 cup water

1. Slice cabbage finely and boil in water with caraway seeds for 5 minutes.
2. Blend tofu, umeboshi plums, and kuzu (mixed in 1/2 cup cold water). Place in pan and bring gently to a boil. Stir well.
3. Pour over cabbage and serve.

140. Fresh Dill Sauce

Serves 4

>1/2 cup fresh dill weed, chopped fine
>1/2 cup rice, soy, or oat milk (unsweetened)
>1 1/2 teaspoons kuzu
>1 cup water
>Pinch of salt

1. Heat the milk and add the dill.
2. Mix kuzu well in water and add to the warm dill and milk, sprinkle in salt.
3. Gently bring to a boil. Serve over fish or Millet-Aduki Croquettes (*see* Recipe 49).

141. Hummus

Serves a party

>3/4 cup chickpeas
>4 cups water
>4 slices kombu, 1" x 2" approx.
>Pinch of salt
>2 tablespoons tahini
>1 tablespoon fresh lemon juice
>2 cloves garlic, crushed
>1/2 cup water
>2 tablespoons umeboshi vinegar
>Chopped parsley, to garnish

1. Wash chickpeas and soak overnight in 2 cups water.
2. Discard water and add 3 cups fresh. Boil in pressure cooker with kombu for 1 1/2 hours or in covered pan for 3 hours, adding more water if necessary.
3. When soft, add salt and boil another 1/2 hour.
4. Blend chickpeas, kombu, and any water left.
5. Place tahini in a pan and heat gently, stirring well, then add the lemon juice and garlic. Add a little water if necessary to keep it from sticking to pan. When it bubbles, remove from heat and add umeboshi vinegar.

6. Stir the tahini into the chickpeas.

7. Garnish with parsley and serve.

142. Guacamole (A Mexican Dip)

Serves a party

>3 ripe avocados
>Juice of 1 lemon
>1 tablespoon tamari
>1 medium red onion, chopped fine
>1 clove garlic, crushed
>2 or 3 drops of Tabasco (hot pepper) sauce (to taste)

1. Peel and pit the avocados. Mash with a fork.

2 Add lemon juice and tamari.

3. Mix the chopped onion, garlic, and Tabasco thoroughly into the mixture.

4. Serve with corn chips.

143. Lemon Sauce

Serves 4

>2 tablespoons whole corn flour
>2 teaspoons safflower oil
>1 cup rice or oat milk
>1 teaspoon soy sauce
>Juice of 1/2 lemon
>1 teaspoon lemon rind
>1 teaspoon kuzu
>1/2 cup cold water

1. Place corn flour in hot oil. Stir.

2. Gently mix in milk.

3. Add soy sauce, lemon juice, and rind.

4. Mix kuzu in cold water. Pour in and stir. Serve over Millet-Arame Croquettes (*see* Recipe 50).

144. Miso and Barley Malt Orange Dip

Dip for 4

>3 tablespoons water
>1 tablespoon barley malt
>2 teaspoons tahini
>1 tablespoon mirin or sake
>1 teaspoon hatcho miso
>1 tablespoon boiling water
>Juice of half an orange
>2 or 3 drops of Tabasco (hot pepper) sauce (to taste)

1. Mix water, barley malt, tahini, and mirin or sake in a heated pan. Using a wooden spoon, stir well. Mixture should be smooth. Add more water if necessary. Turn off heat.

2. Mix miso in 1 tablespoon boiling water, then add orange juice and 3 drops Tabasco sauce. Stir into the tahini sauce. Serve as a dip with Prawns and Sesame Toast (*see* Recipe 174).

145. Miso Dressing for Salads

> 1 level teaspoon natto miso
> 1 level teaspoon genmai or buckwheat miso
> 1/2 cup boiling water
> 1 teaspoon olive oil
> 1 teaspoon rice vinegar

1. Mix misos with water.
2. Add olive oil and vinegar.
3. Stir well and serve over salads.

146. Mochi and Onion Sauce

Mochi is made from cooked, pounded, sweet rice (*see* INGREDIENTS—Mochi).

> 1 1/2 cups water
> 1 medium onion, diced
> 3/4 cup grated mochi
> 2 teaspoons light tahini
> 1 tablespoon umeboshi vinegar
> 1 tablespoon juice of fresh grated ginger (optional)

1. Bring water to a boil and add onion. Simmer for 5 minutes.
2. Add grated mochi and stir well until sauce thickens.
3. Add tahini, umeboshi vinegar, and ginger. Stir and remove from heat.
4. Serve over buckwheat burgers or rice croquettes.

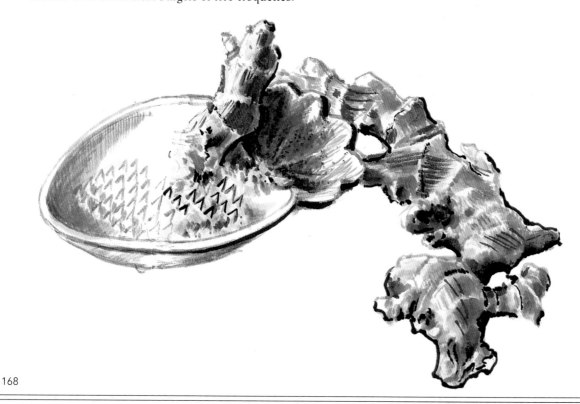

147. Mochi-Umeboshi "Mock Cheese" Sauce

Serves 4 to 6

> 3 cups water
> 1 medium onion, sliced fine (1 cup)
> 1 teaspoon light tahini
> 1 teaspoon caraway seeds or basil
> 3/4 cup grated mochi
> 1 teaspoon white miso
> 1/2 cup hot water
> 1 teaspoon umeboshi vinegar

1. Bring water to a boil in a pot. Add onion and simmer 3 minutes.
2. Add tahini, caraway seeds or basil, and grated mochi. Stir well.
3. Mix the miso in water to a smooth consistency. Add to the sauce and stir.
4. Add the umeboshi vinegar and stir. The "cheese" sauce is ready.
5. Serve over Aduki Pizza (*see* Recipe 130) or Aduki Rice and Sweet Corn Croquettes (*see* Recipe 131) or with noodles.

148. Mushroom and Pepper Sauce with Ginger and Kuzu

Serves 4 to 6

> 3 cups water
> 1 teaspoon grated ginger
> 1/2 red pepper
> 2 large mushrooms, diced
> 1/2 cup tamari
> 2 teaspoons kuzu
> 1/2 cup water

1. Bring water to a boil with ginger.
2. Place red pepper under a medium grill until skin is charred and can be easily removed. Slice remaining flesh into small pieces. Add with mushrooms to ginger water. Simmer for 5 minutes.
3. Add tamari.
4. Dissolve kuzu in 1/2 cup of water, add to mixture, and stir until it thickens to a smooth sauce.
5. Serve over grains or noodles.

149. Nori Spread

Serves 2 to 4

> 4 sheets nori cut small, 1/4" squares
> 3/4 cup hot water
> 2 teaspoons olive oil
> 2 teaspoons umeboshi vinegar
> 2 teaspoons tamari
> 2 teaspoons mirin
> 2 teaspoons kuzu mixed in 1/2 cup cold water

1. Place nori in small pan over medium heat. Using small wooden spoon, stir briskly for 2 to 3 minutes.

2. Add olive oil. Stir 1 minute.

3. Lower heat, add hot water, tamari, umeboshi, miren, and kuzu in water. Stir until it blends and sets to a paste (but don't boil). Cool and serve.

Use spread with a squeeze of lemon or on bannocks with hummus and pressed salad. Store in refrigerator.

150. Oatmeal Sauce

Serves 4

> 1 tablespoon whole wheat flour
> 1 tablespoon oat flakes
> 3 cups water (or vegetable water)
> 1 pinch kombu powder
> 1 tablespoon grated ginger
> 1 tablespoon umeboshi vinegar
> Bread crumbs

1. Mix flour and oat flakes in water. Sprinkle with kombu and bring to a boil.

2. Add ginger and umeboshi vinegar, stirring well. Add more water if necessary.

3. Pour sauce over Stuffed Cabbage (*see* Recipe 42) and sprinkle with bread crumbs. Brown in oven for 5 minutes or so and serve.

151. Onion and Squash Sauce

Serves 4 to 6

> 1 Spanish onion, finely chopped
> 2 regular onions, finely chopped
> 1/2 teaspoon sesame oil
> 1/2 teaspoon corn oil
> 1 teaspoon grated ginger
> 1 teaspoon tekka condiment
> 2 cups baked pumpkin or butternut squash
> 2 tablespoons tamari
> 1 cup water

1. Sauté onions in oil, stirring for 5 minutes over low heat.

2. Add ginger and tekka. Simmer another 20 minutes.

3. Blend baked pumpkin or squash with tamari and 1 cup water.

4. Add squash to onions, bring to a boil, and simmer gently for 25 minutes. Add more water if needed.

5. Serve over Millet-Aduki Croquettes (*see* Recipe 49), Buckwheat Burgers (*see* Recipe 39) or soba noodles (*see* INGREDIENTS—Noodles).

152. Pesto Sauce

Serves 4 to 6

2 cups fresh basil
1 clove garlic, sliced
1 cup water
1 teaspoon light shiro miso
1/2 cup hot water
2 tablespoons olive oil
2 tablespoons roasted pine nuts

1. Blend basil and garlic with 1 cup water and place in pan.

2. Mix miso in hot water and add the oil. Blend.

3. Add roasted pine nuts to miso liquid and blend.

4. Bring basil and garlic to a boil. Simmer for 2 minutes only. Add miso mixture and remove from heat just before it boils.

5. Serve with brown rice udon noodles (*see* INGREDIENTS—Noodles).

153. Salad Dressing: Apple Juice and Tamari

Serves 6
An "oil and vinegar" dressing.

3/4 cup apple juice
1 tablespoon sesame oil
1 teaspoon tamari
1 umeboshi plum (pitted and sliced) or 2 teaspoons umeboshi vinegar
1/2 teaspoon sesame salt (*see* INGREDIENTS—Sesame Seeds)

1. Mix apple juice, sesame oil, and tamari and add umeboshi.

2. Sprinkle on sesame salt and serve over salad.

154. Sweet and Sour Barley Malt and Ginger Sauce

Serves 4

2 teaspoons brown rice vinegar
2 teaspoons tamari
2 teaspoons brown (roasted) sesame oil
2 teaspoons barley malt
2 teaspoons ginger juice
1 teaspoon roasted sesame seeds
3/4 cup water

1. Warm brown rice vinegar, tamari, and sesame oil in a pan over low heat, mixing well.

2. Stir in barley malt, ginger juice, sesame seeds, and water.

3. Serve over swordfish or other fish and top with small ginger slices.
This sauce can also be served with chicken.

155. Sweet and Sour Sauce with Mushrooms and Scallions

Serves 4 to 6

> 2 tablespoons sweet brown rice vinegar
> 4 teaspoons barley malt
> 1 tablespoon tamari
> 1 cup water
> 1 scallion, chopped
> 2 mushrooms, sliced
> 1/4 red pepper, finely sliced
> 1 teaspoon kuzu
> 1/2 cup water

1. Heat vinegar and stir in barley malt and tamari.
2. Add the cup of water and bring almost to a boil.
3. Blacken pepper over flame and peel. Slice fine.
4. Add vegetables and simmer 2 minutes.
5. Mix kuzu well in half cup of water and add to mixture; stir until it thickens. Remove from heat.
6. Serve over fish.

156. Tahini, Ginger, and Scallion Miso Spread

A spread for 4

> 1 tablespoon fresh ginger juice
> 1 scallion, finely sliced
> 1 teaspoon toasted sesame oil
> 1/2 cup tahini
> 1 cup water
> 2 teaspoons white miso
> 1/2 cup boiling water or vegetable water

1. Roast ginger and scallion in the sesame oil for 2 minutes over low heat.
2. Add tahini and water and stir constantly until it bubbles. Remove from heat.
3. Mix miso in boiling water and add to the spread; mix thoroughly. Allow to cool.
4. Refrigerate after use. Add a little water and stir each time before serving. Good on bannocks or bread, toast or rice cakes. Can also be mixed with 1 tablespoon soft, cooked whole oats.

157. Tahini, Lemon, and Tamari Dressing

Serves 4

> 1 tablespoon tahini
> Juice of 1 lemon
> 1/2 cup boiling water or vegetable water
> 1 tablespoon tamari
> 1 tablespoon chopped dill or parsley

1. Mix tahini and lemon.

2. Slowly add the water until smooth.

3. Add tamari and dill or parsley.

4. Serve with salad or over rice.

158. Tahini and Soy Sauce

Serves 4 to 6

> 2 tablespoons tahini
> 1 tablespoon tamari
> 1 cup water or vegetable water
> 1 teaspoon kuzu
> 1/2 cup cold water

1. Mix the tahini and soy sauce in a small saucepan.

2. Add the water and heat gently. Stir.

3. Mix kuzu in cold water and add to the mixture.

4. Bring almost to a boil, until mixture becomes creamy.

5. Serve over croquettes or rice, fish or tempeh (*see* Recipe 134).

159. Tahini, Rice Vinegar, and Miso Dressing

Serves 4

> 1 tablespoon tahini
> 1 tablespoon light shiro miso
> 1 tablespoon rice vinegar
> 1/2 cup water

1. Heat tahini gently until it bubbles. Remove from heat.

2. Mix tahini with white miso and rice vinegar.

3. Add water to the mixture—this should be a fairly thick dressing. Serve on salad.

160. Tofu Cheese

> 1 teaspoon genmai rice miso
> 1 teaspoon light shiro miso
> 2 tablespoons boiling water
> 1 half-pound block tofu

1. Mix misos with water.

2. Cover the tofu surface with the miso.

3. Leave to ferment at room temperature for 2 days.

4. Add chopped herbs (chives, tarragon, etc.) if desired. Delicious served with hot bread, toast, or crackers.

161. Tofu-Dill Salad Spread

Serves 4 to 6

>1/2 green pepper
>2 cups diced tofu
>1 tablespoon chopped celery
>1 tablespoon chopped dill-salted pickles (*see* Recipe 114)
>1 tablespoon lemon juice
>1 teaspoon safflower oil
>1 tablespoon umeboshi vinegar
>1 tablespoon chopped dill
>1/2 teaspoon natural mustard
>Pinch of salt

1. Grill pepper or heat over flame until skin can be easily peeled away. Chop flesh finely.

2. Blend ingredients together and serve with bannocks, whole wheat bread, or sesame crackers.

162. Tofu Sauce Tartare

>2 tablespoons tofu
>1/2 cup water
>3 teaspoons fresh ginger juice
>2 umeboshi plums, pitted and crushed
>1/2 cup oat or rice milk
>1 tablespoon safflower mayonnaise (optional)
>1/2 cup finely chopped, fresh scallions or chives or 1 pickled cucumber chopped,
>   (*see* Recipe 114)

1. Parboil tofu in water for 5 minutes.

2. Blend tofu in a suribachi with ginger juice and umeboshi.

3. Add milk and mayonnaise (optional). Mix to a creamy consistency.

4. Add scallions, chives, or pickled cucumber, and serve with fish.

163. Umeboshi and Kuzu Sauce

Serves 4

>1 cup water
>1 pinch kombu powder
>1 medium onion, diced
>2 tablespoons umeboshi vinegar
>1 teaspoon kuzu
>1/2 cup cold water
>1 tablespoon mirin
>1/4 cup chopped parsley

1. Bring water and kombu to a boil. Add onion and sauté for 4 minutes.

2. Add umeboshi vinegar and simmer for 1 minute.

3. Mix kuzu in water and add to the mixture with mirin and parsley. Stir until sauce thickens.

4. Serve over vegetables or cooked, chopped vegetables can be added to it and it can be served with rice or noodles.

164. Umeboshi-Mustard Sauce

Serves 4

> 2 teaspoons natural or Dijon mustard
> 1/2 tablespoon umeboshi paste or 2 umeboshi plums, pitted and mashed
> 1 cup vegetable water
> 1 teaspoon kuzu
> 1 tablespoon arrowroot
> 2 teaspoons tamari
> 1/2 cup cold water

1. Mix mustard and umeboshi in vegetable water and heat gently in a pan.

2. Mix kuzu, arrowroot, and tamari in cold water and add to the pan. Simmer for 3 minutes, stirring well. Add a little more water if necessary to make sauce and add to Prawns with Lotus Root (Recipe 175).

If using mustard powder, mix it with a little umeboshi vinegar.

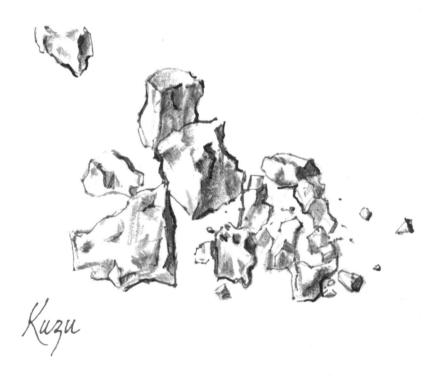

Kuzu

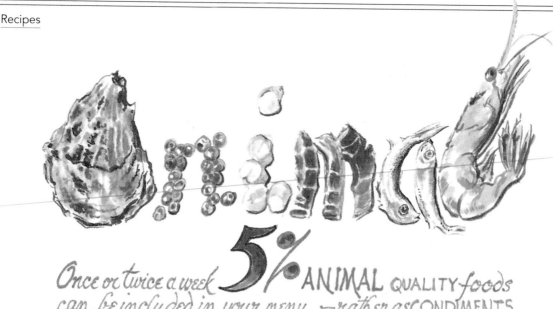

animal

5%

Once or twice a week **ANIMAL** quality *foods* can be included in your menu — rather as CONDIMENTS. Shell fish, fish (cooked or eaten RAW), wild or free range birds are preferred to MAMMAL meats (pork, beef etc.) which are usually CHEMICALLY produced or treated. Always serve with VEGETABLES and GRAINS for balance.

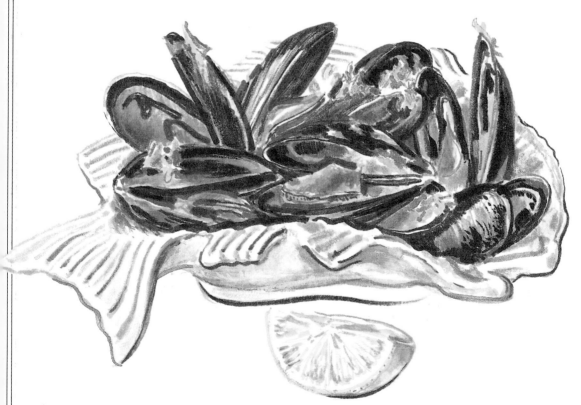

Animal Products

165. Chicken and Cashew Nuts in Sweet and Sour Sauce

Serves 6 to 8

>4 boneless and skinless free-range chicken breast filets
>3/4 cup cashew nuts
>1 tablespoon toasted sesame oil
>2 cups water
>2 cups apple juice
>1 tablespoon barley or rice malt syrup
>1 tablespoon tamari
>1 tablespoon umeboshi vinegar
>1 tablespoon mirin
>2 teaspoons kuzu in 1/2 cup apple juice

1. Place the chicken breasts with the nuts in an oiled pan. Sauté for 5 minutes.
2. Pour in water and apple juice, barley malt, tamari, umeboshi vinegar, and mirin. Stir. Lower heat. Simmer 35 minutes.
3. Mix kuzu in 1/2 cup apple juice. Add to the mixture and stir. Remove from heat before mixture boils.
4. Serve with brown rice and vegetables.

166. Chicken and Mango Roast

Serves 6 to 8

>8 slices dried mango
>3/4 cup water
>4 free-range chicken breast filets
>2 cups cranberry juice
>2 tablespoons tamari

1. Preheat oven to 400°F/200°C.
2. Soak mango in water for 10 minutes.
3. Remove any fat from chicken and place chicken in a shallow baking dish.
4. Pour cranberry juice and a little tamari over the chicken.
5. Place 2 mango slices on each portion and pour in water from soaking mango.
6. Cook in preheated oven for 30 minutes, turn pieces, and cook another 20 minutes.

Fresh mango or any dried fruit such as apricot can be used.

167. Chicken in Béchamel Sauce with Grapes

Serves 4

>2 free-range chicken breasts, skinned
>3 cups water
>1 pinch salt
>1 small carrot, sliced
>1 small onion, sliced
>1 stalk celery, sliced fine
>1/2 cup chopped parsley
>2 teaspoons kuzu
>1/2 cup oat milk
>1 cup seedless green grapes
>1 tablespoon sake or dry white wine (optional)

1. Bring water to a boil, add chicken and salt. Simmer over medium heat for 10 minutes.
2. Add sliced vegetables. Simmer over low heat for 20 minutes or until chicken is tender.
3. Remove chicken from stock and slice into small pieces. Return to pot.
4. Mix kuzu in milk then add to the chicken and vegetables. Stir until sauce thickens.
5. Add grapes and sake or white wine.
6. Serve with hot rice.

168. Cod Filets with Miso, Shallot, and Scallion Sauce

Serves 4

>1 1/2 pounds cod
>2 teaspoons light miso
>Juice of 1 lemon
>2 teaspoons sesame oil
>1 large shallot, diagonally sliced
>1 clove garlic, crushed
>2 sliced scallions
>8 snow peas
>2 tablespoons fresh, chopped dill
>Parsley, to garnish

1. Slice cod into filets. Remove back skin.
2. Mix miso and lemon juice.
3. Place oil in a pan and heat. Sauté shallot, garlic, and half of scallion for 2 to 3 minutes over medium heat.
4. Add cod filets, the rest of the scallion, snow peas, and dill. Pour on the miso and lemon. Cover and cook for 10 minutes.
5. Garnish with parsley and serve with brown rice.

169. Crab and Sweet Corn Soup

Serves 4

  4 cups water
  1 pinch kombu powder
  2 fresh ears of corn
  1 cup sliced, fresh, cooked crab pieces
  1 tablespoon kuzu
  3/4 cup cold oat or rice milk
  Pinch of salt
  1/4 cup freshly chopped parsley

1. Bring water with kombu to a boil and cook ears of corn for 10 minutes. Remove kernels and keep water.

2. Place corn kernels and crab meat in corn water. Bring to a boil and simmer 2 minutes.

3. Mix the kuzu in the milk and add to the soup to thicken it. Heat until liquid clears.

4. Add pinch of salt. Stir.

5. Decorate with parsley and serve. One or two drops of tamari can be added to taste.

170. Fish "Bouillabaisse" Soup

Serves 6 to 8

  8 cups water
  1 slice kombu, 2"x 4"
  2 cups salmon pieces
  2 cups white fish
  1 cup squid, cleaned and sliced in rings
  2 bay leaves
  6 coriander seeds, ground fine
  Pinch of salt
  1 tablespoon sesame oil
  2 medium onions, sliced fine
  1 clove garlic, crushed
  1/2 red pepper
  1 small leek, sliced fine
  1/2 teaspoon saffron powder
  8 cooked prawns
  2 teaspoons kuzu
  1 cup water
  3 slices whole wheat bread pan-toasted in 1 teaspoon of olive oil

1. Bring water to a boil with kombu. Simmer for 3 minutes. Remove kombu, slice it into 1/4" squares, and return to water.

2. Add salmon, white fish, squid, bay leaves, coriander seeds, and salt. Simmer for 15 to 20 minutes. When fish is tender, remove it, take out bones, and return to the soup.

3. Blacken a red pepper over a flame and remove the skin. Cut flesh into 1/2" squares. Heat oil in a pan and add onions, garlic, red pepper, leek, and saffron. Sauté for 5 to 8 minutes.

4. Mix fish and vegetables and add the prawns. Simmer for 25 minutes.

5. Mix kuzu in water and add to the soup. Stir until it thickens.

6. Slice pan-toasted bread into 1/2" squares and serve with the soup.

179

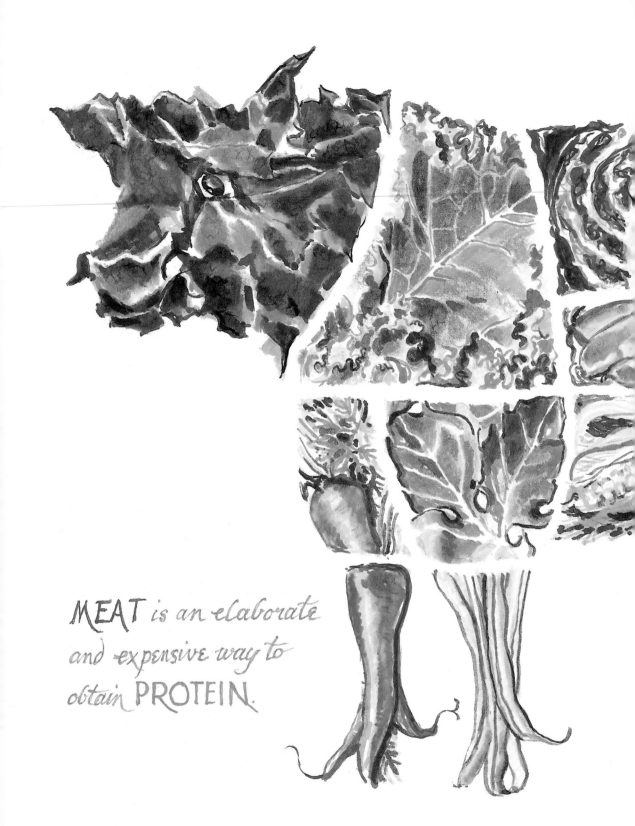

MEAT is an elaborate and expensive way to obtain PROTEIN.

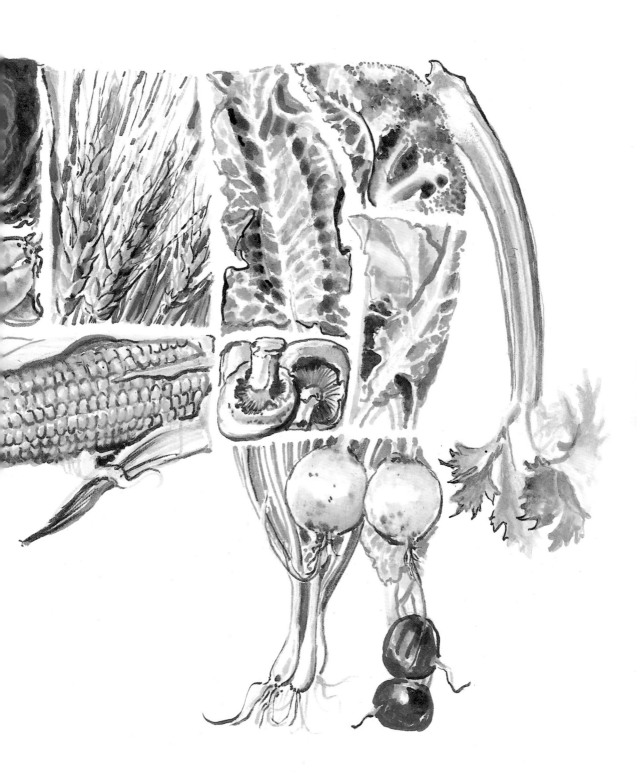

171. New England Fish Chowder with Cream of Tahini

Serves 4 to 6

1 tablespoon olive oil
1 clove garlic, chopped
1 medium onion, sliced
2 pinches salt
1/4 pound dark fish (bluefish or mackerel or tuna)
1/4 cup carrot pieces
1/4 cup sliced turnip
1/4 cup red pepper pieces (roast skin over flame to remove)
1/4 cup celery pieces
1/4 teaspoon basil
4 cups water to cover
1/4 pound white fish (sole or haddock)
1/2 cup rice flour
1 teaspoon tahini
1 cup water
1/4 cup chopped parsley

1. Heat olive oil in pot over medium heat. Don't let it get too hot.
2. Add garlic to oil and sauté for 2 minutes.
3. Add sliced onion and salt. Stir well. Cover after 2 minutes and cook another 7 minutes.
4. Slice dark fish in small chunks. Add to onions and stir. Cook for 5 minutes.
5. Add carrots, turnip, red pepper flesh, celery, and basil. Cook 5–10 minutes.
6. Cover with water and cook 10 more minutes.
7. Add white fish chunks and cook another 15 minutes.
8. Mix rice flour and tahini with enough water to make a creamy paste. Add this to cream the soup.
9. Decorate with chopped parsley and serve.

172. Paella

Serves 4 to 6

3 cups brown rice
6 cups water
1 tablespoon olive oil
2 large onions, finely sliced
1 clove garlic, crushed
1/2 teaspoon saffron powder or turmeric
1/2 red pepper, sliced (roast skin over flame to remove)
6 pieces chicken meat
2 pinches of salt
4 cups water
6 scrubbed mussels (closed when fresh)
6 large prawns in their shells
1 cup fresh, sliced squid
1 cup fresh green beans or 1 cup fresh green peas
1/2 cup water

1 cup fresh, chopped parsley
1 lemon (sliced)

1. Cook the rice in 6 cups water over medium heat until water is absorbed (30 minutes). The rice should not be completely cooked.

2. Heat oil in heavy pan or skillet and sauté onions and garlic for 2 minutes.

3. Add saffron or turmeric, red pepper, chicken, and a pinch of salt. Sauté and stir well for 10 minutes over low heat.

4. Add 2 cups water and simmer for 15 minutes, or until chicken is tender.

5. Preheat oven to 300°F/150°C.

6. Mix the rice and the chicken mixture in a shallow ovenproof dish.

7. Bring remaining 2 cups of water to a boil. Add remaining salt and drop in mussels, prawns, and squid. Boil over high heat for 5 minutes. Mussels should open.

8. Decorate rice and chicken with the various shellfish and squid and pour remaining fish water over it.

9. Cover paella well with a lid or foil and place in preheated oven for 25 minutes, or until liquid is absorbed and the rice soft.

10. Cook beans (or peas) in water gently for 5 minutes (until water has evaporated).

11. Decorate paella with beans (or peas), parsley and lemon slices and serve.

Note: Paella can be made using diced tofu as well as or instead of chicken.

173. Pheasant Casserole

Serves 4

1 tablespoon corn oil or sesame oil
2 medium onions, sliced
1 pheasant (plucked and cleaned)
1 apple, sliced
1 cup chopped parsley
1 cup fresh cranberries or 1/2 cup raisins
Pinch of salt
1 bay leaf
Pinch of coriander
2 cloves
2 cups apple juice
2 teaspoons arrowroot
1/2 cup water
1/2 cup red wine (or to taste)

1. Preheat oven to 300°F/150°C.

2. Heat a heavy casserole over medium heat. Add oil.

3. Sauté onions with the pheasant, apple, parsley, cranberries (or raisins), pinch of salt, bay leaf, coriander, and cloves. Stir ingredients well for 10 minutes.

4. Add apple juice.

5. Cover and place in preheated oven for 1 hour.

6. If gravy needs thickening, mix arrowroot in water and add to the casserole with red wine before serving.

7. Serve with rice, Red Cabbage (*see* Recipe 120) and Parsnips and Onion (*see* Recipe 112).

Beware of steel shot when eating pheasant!

174. Prawns and Sesame Toast

Serves 4 to 6

> 8 jumbo prawns (shrimp)
> 1 teaspoon kuzu
> 1/2 cup rice milk or water
> 1 tablespoon whole wheat flour
> 1 teaspoon rice flour
> 1 teaspoon corn flour
> 1 pinch salt
> 1/2 scallion, finely chopped
> 1 teaspoon fresh ginger, grated
> 2 slices whole wheat bread
> 2 tablespoons olive oil
> 2 tablespoons sesame seeds
> 1 lemon, sliced

1. Shell and wash prawns. Place in a medium bowl. Mash well with ginger and scallion.
2. Stir kuzu in the milk or water. Add flours and stir to make a not-too-wet paste.
3. Pour onto prawns and mix to make a spread. Let stand for 20 minutes or more.
4. Cut the bread into quarters. Spread the prawn mixture on the one side. Sprinkle sesame seeds over and firmly press them onto the surface.
5. Heat oil in flat pan or wok. Gently place each spread surface face down and cook for 2 to 3 minutes. When golden brown, turn over and fry the bread base. Quarter slices and serve with Tahini, Lemon, and Tamari Dressing (*see* Recipe 157).

175. Prawns with Lotus Root and Umeboshi-Mustard Sauce

Serves 2

> 1 teaspoon toasted sesame oil
> 1 cup fresh lotus root, sliced fine or 1 cup diced lotus root, soaked in water for 1/2 hour (keep water)
> 1 clove garlic, finely chopped
> 2 scallions, sliced diagonally
> 6 large prawns (shrimp), sliced
> 1 cup fresh snow peas

1. Place oil in preheated iron skillet, add lotus root, garlic, and half the scallions. Simmer over medium heat and stir well for 10 minutes.
2. Add prawns and rest of the scallions. Simmer another 10 minutes. Add snow peas and stir for 2 minutes.
3. Serve with Umeboshi-Mustard Sauce (*see* Recipe 164).

176. Prawns with Mochi-Lemon Sauce

Serves 4

> 3 cups water
> 1 large onion, finely chopped
> 4 teaspoons tahini
> Juice of 1/2 lemon

2 teaspoons fresh lemon rind
1 tablespoon tamari
3/4 cup grated mochi
12 small prawns (shrimp)

1. Bring water to a boil. Add onion and simmer 10 minutes over low heat.

2. Add tahini, lemon juice and rind, and tamari.

3. Add prawns. Stir for 2 minutes.

4. Add grated mochi and stir until sauce is smooth.

5. Serve on noodles or whole wheat spaghetti.

177. Salmon Roe and Avocado

Serves 4

2 avocados
1/3 cup pressed salad (see Recipe 117)
1 small onion, finely chopped
3 teaspoons salmon roe "caviar" or lump fish "caviar"
1 pitted umeboshi plum, sliced into four sections
Chopped parsley to garnish
1 lemon

1. Slice avocados in half. Remove pits.

2. Place a teaspoon of salad and chopped onion in each.

3. Drop in 1/2 teaspoon salmon roe and top it with 1/4 slice of umeboshi.

4. Serve garnished with 1/4 of a lemon, chopped parsley, and Salad Dressing (*see* Recipe 153).
Good eaten with hot bannocks—Recipe 69—and hummus—Recipe 141.

178. Scallops with Rice or Noodles

Serves 4

1 teaspoon corn oil
1 small onion, diced
1/2 clove garlic, finely chopped
1 cup small scallops
1 teaspoon kuzu
1 teaspoon corn flour
3/4 cup oat or rice milk
1/2 cup water (more or less)
1/4 cup chopped parsley
1 tablespoon sake or white wine (optional)

1. Heat oil in iron skillet or pan. Add onion and garlic. Stir-fry for 5 minutes.

2. Add scallops. Stir-fry for 3 minutes.

3. Dissolve kuzu in milk.

4. Mix kuzu and corn flour in cold milk. Pour over scallops, onions, and garlic. Stir well until sauce thickens. Add a little more water if needed. Add half the parsley with sake or wine.

5. Stir and serve over rice or noodles. Decorate with rest of parsley.

179. Sukiyaki, Udon Noodles, and Seafood

Serves 4

This dish can be cooked in the kitchen or using a hot plate at the table.

THE BROTH

> 4 cups udon noodles, cooked and strained (*see* INGREDIENTS—Noodles)
> 6 cups kombu and shiitake mushroom broth with tamari (*see* INGREDIENTS—Dashi)

THE SEAFOOD

> 6 scallops
> 6 clams in their shells (scrubbed)
> 8 shrimp
> 1 cup watercress (washed)
> 8 fresh mushrooms
> 4 scallions, finely sliced diagonally
> 4 Chinese cabbage leaves, sliced into 1/2" pieces
> Sliced lemon

1. Heat dashi or noodle broth in the iron skillet (a little can be placed in small side dishes to use as a dipping sauce).

2. Arrange the seafood decoratively in the broth, adding them according to the time they take to cook. Simmer 5 to 10 minutes.

3. Serve with slices of lemon.

180. Swordfish with Tarragon

Serves 4

> 1 pound swordfish
> 1/2 teaspoon white miso
> 1/2 teaspoon mugi miso
> 1/4 cup hot water
> Juice of 1/2 lemon
> 1 teaspoon fresh, chopped tarragon or 1 1/2 teaspoons diced tarragon

1. Preheat oven to 375°F/190°C.

2. Place fish in ovenproof dish.

3. Mix misos with hot water and squeeze in lemon juice.

4. Sprinkle chopped tarragon on fish and pour miso and lemon over it.

5. Bake in preheated oven for 1/2 hour.

6. Serve. Good with boiled millet and Tahini and Soy Sauce (*see* Recipe 158).

183. Turkey Croquettes and Onion Sauce

Makes 4 to 6 croquettes

>2 cups finely chopped cooked turkey meat
>1 onion, chopped
>1 cup chopped parsley
>1 tablespoon mugi miso
>1/2 cup warm water
>1 tablespoon fresh, grated ginger
>1 1/2 cups soft, cooked brown rice (*see* INGREDIENTS—Grains)
>1 cup oatmeal
>1 cup bread crumbs (or oatmeal)
>1 tablespoon corn oil

1. Preheat oven to 350°F/180°C.

2. Mix the turkey, onion, and parsley.

3. Mix miso in warm water and add to the turkey mixture with the ginger.

4. Add cooked rice and oatmeal and mix.

5. Wet hands and roll croquettes in bread crumbs (or oatmeal).

6. Pan-fry over gentle heat for 3 minutes on each side.

7. Place in preheated oven for 1/2 hour and serve with Onion or Parsley Béchamel Sauce (*see* variations of Recipe 137).

Can also be made with salmon.

182. Wakame and Shrimp Soup

Serves 4

>1/2 cup soaked wakame
>1 cup soaking water
>4 cups water
>6 or 8 shrimp, sliced
>1 tablespoon tamari
>1 scallion, diagonally sliced
>4 slices lemon

1. Slice wakame into very small slices. They will expand, so do this thoroughly. Place in a pan with the soaking water.

2. Add water. Bring to boil and then simmer 10 minutes.

3. Add the shrimp and tamari and simmer another 10 minutes.

4. Sprinkle with scallion and serve with a 1/2 slice of lemon for each bowl.

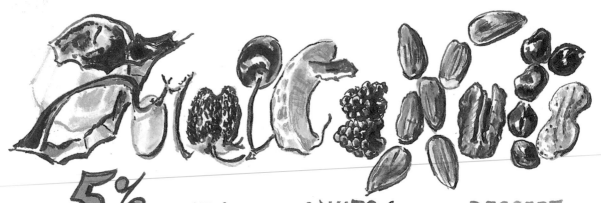

Fruit & Nuts

5% FRUIT *in season* & NUTS *for your* DESSERT
which can include GRAINS & GRAIN PRODUCTS *(pastry,*
cakes, puddings, cereals, sweet rice) sweet VEGETABLES
such as **carrots, pumpkin, squash** — *even Azuki Beans.*
AGAR, CARRAGEEN, KUZU & TOFU *for jellies & whips.*

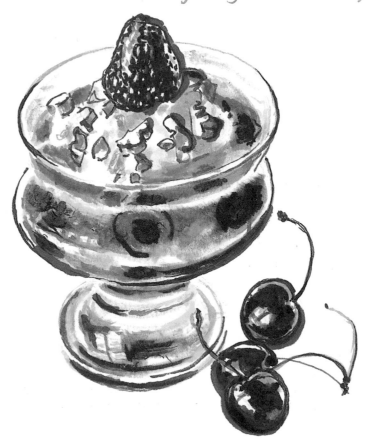

Desserts

183. Almond Cream

Topping for 4

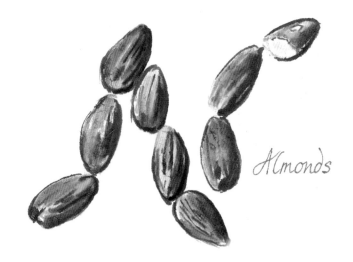

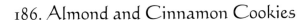

1 cup peeled almonds
1 1/4 cups oat or rice milk
1 tablespoon corn syrup
1 drop vanilla extract

1. Grind almonds in an electric blender.
2. Add milk, corn syrup, and vanilla and blend until creamy. (Add more milk if necessary.) Refrigerate.
3. Serve as a cream over kanten and top with strawberries or cherries, or sprinkled with grated nuts.

Amazake milk can be used instead of soy milk and corn syrup.

186. Almond and Cinnamon Cookies

Makes 12 small cookies

1 1/4 cups whole wheat pastry flour
1/4 teaspoon cinnamon
2 tablespoons corn or sesame oil
2 cups slivered or flaked almonds
1 tablespoon rice syrup or barley malt
1/2 cup apple juice (more or less)
1 tablespoon apple and pear spread or other sugarless jam (optional)

1. Preheat oven to 350°F/180°C.
2. Mix flour with cinnamon and stir in oil.
3. Add almonds with rice syrup. Stir well.
4. Use enough apple juice to make a soft, not-too-wet, mix.
5. Place small cookie shapes on an oiled, lightly floured, baking sheet and press a small indentation on top of each one. Drop in 1/4 teaspoon sugarless jam.
6. Bake in a preheated oven on a low rack for 10 minutes. Turn heat down to 300° F and bake for 30 minutes.
7. If using apple and pear spread, place another small quantity on top of each and bake another 5 minutes before taking out of the oven so that spread will set.

185. Amazake and Pear "Blancmange"

Serves 4

> 2 cups amazake milk (*see* INGREDIENTS—Amazake)
> 2 teaspoons kuzu
> 1 cup apple juice
> 1 pear, sliced
> 2 tablespoons cashew nuts

1. Heat amazake gently in a pan.

2. Mix kuzu in the cold apple juice and add to amazake. Stir until it thickens and begins to boil.

3. Place pear slices into dessert dishes and pour amazake cream over them.

4. Roast nuts in iron skillet. Chop fine and sprinkle over the top of the amazake.

5. Cool and refrigerate before serving. Serve with a dollop of Tofu Cream Whip (*see* Recipe 220). Blackberries can be used instead of the pear. Keep four to decorate the top. This can also be made by substituting 2 cups soy milk and 2 teaspoons barley malt or rice syrup for the amazake milk.

186. Amazake Kanten with Almonds and Strawberries

Serves 6

> 4 cups amazake milk (*see* INGREDIENTS—Amazake)
> 2 teaspoons agar-agar flakes
> 2 drops almond extract
> 1/2 cup chopped, roasted almonds
> 6 fresh strawberries

1. Heat amazake. Add agar-agar and almond extract. Bring to a boil.

2. Pour into a bowl or into separate containers.

3. Sprinkle with chopped almonds and top with strawberries.

This can also be made by substituting 4 cups oat milk and 1 tablespoon barley malt for the amazake.

187. Apple and Blackberry or Peach Crumble

Serves 4 to 6

1 cup whole wheat flour
1 1/2 cups rolled oats (uncooked)
1/2 teaspoon salt
1/2 teaspoon cinnamon
1/4 cup sesame oil
1 teaspoon fresh, grated lemon rind
1/4 cup water
2 cups sliced apples
1/2 cup apple juice
2 cups blackberries or 2 cups sliced peaches
1 teaspoon sesame oil
1 tablespoon barley malt syrup (optional)

1. Preheat oven to 350°F/180°C.
2. To make crumble mixture, mix dry ingredients and add sesame oil, lemon rind, and water. Stir well.
3. Apples should be peeled first (unless they are organically grown). Boil them in the apple juice for 5 minutes over low heat.
4. Mix with the blackberries or peaches.
5. Oil a shallow pie pan and pour in fruit.
6. Sprinkle crumble over the fruit and pour barley malt syrup over the mixture.
7. Place in preheated oven for 35 minutes.

188. Apple and Cinnamon Kanten Dessert

Serves 2 to 4

2 cups water
2 apples, sliced
1 tablespoon raisins
1/2 teaspoon cinnamon
Pinch of salt
1 teaspoon kuzu
1 cup apple juice
2 teaspoons barley malt syrup
1 1/2 teaspoons agar-agar flakes

1. Bring water to a boil and add apples, raisins, cinnamon, and salt. Simmer gently for 5 minutes, or until apples are soft.
2. Mix kuzu well in apple juice.
3. Add kuzu and barley malt syrup to apples. Stir well over low heat.
4. Sprinkle in the agar-agar flakes and stir well.
5. Wet mold or Pyrex dish and pour in kanten. Let set. Refrigerate for 30 minutes.

This can also be made with apples and hunza (dried) apricots and a variety of fruits.

189. Apple "Fan" Fritters with Barley Malt Sauce

Serves 4

> 2 tablespoons kuzu
> 2 cups cold mineral water
> Pinch of salt
> 2/3 cup 85 percent whole wheat pastry flour
> 1/3 cup cornmeal (maize flour)
> 6 small, sweet apples

1. Mix kuzu in cold water with pinch of salt.
2. Mix pastry flour, salt, and cornmeal (maize flour). Add kuzu water gently. Batter mixture should not be too runny. Let stand 1/2 hour.
3. Cut apples into quarters and remove cores, leaving some skin at one end.
4. Slice each quarter lengthwise into four slices. The skin should hold the slices together. Then gently fan out the slices without breaking the skin.
5. Dip the apple "fans" into the batter to cover and deep-fry (*see* INGREDIENTS—Tempura). Serve with Barley Malt Sauce.

BARLEY MALT SAUCE

> 1 teaspoon kuzu
> 1 cup apple juice
> 2 teaspoons barley malt syrup
> 1/2 teaspoon miso
> 2 teaspoons grated ginger

1. Mix kuzu in 1 tablespoon of the apple juice.
2. Heat rest of apple juice with barley malt syrup, miso, and ginger. Stir and gently bring to a boil.
3. Add kuzu and apple juice and bring to boil.
4. Pour over fritters to glaze.

190. Apple (or Pear) Tart

> 3 to 4 medium sweet apples or pears (peeled and sliced)
> 1 teaspoon kuzu
> 1 cup apple juice
> 1 teaspoon agar-agar flakes
> 2 teaspoons barley malt or 1 tablespoon rice syrup (to taste)
> 1 tablespoon ground almonds
> Pie crust (*see* Recipe 75)

1. Preheat oven to 375°F/190°C.
2. Place pastry in tart pan and sprinkle with almonds. Bake for 10 minutes.
3. Arrange apple (or pear) slices on the pie crust and bake for 20 minutes.
4. Remove from oven and allow to cool.
5. Dissolve the kuzu in the apple juice and heat gently; add barley malt or rice syrup and sprinkle in agar-agar, stirring until it thickens, to make a glaze. Remove from heat just before it boils.
6. Pour over the cool apples or pears.
7. Let set for 1 hour before serving.

191. Apple Juice and Pine Nut Kanten

Serves 4

>3 cups natural apple juice
>1/2 teaspoon cinnamon
>2 tablespoons raisins
>1 tablespoon roasted pine nuts
>2 teaspoons agar-agar flakes

1. Heat apple juice with cinnamon, raisins, and roasted pine nuts for 2 minutes.

2. Stir in agar-agar to dissolve and bring to a boil.

3. Pour into wet mold or separate containers and allow to cool, then refrigerate for 30 minutes.

4. Decorate with Tofutti Cream (*see* Recipe 222).

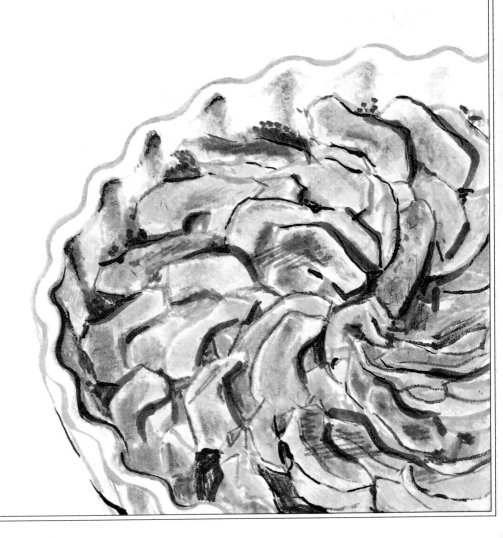

192. Apple and Nut Kanten

Serves 4

2 apples
1 tablespoon seedless raisins
1 cup water
Pinch of salt
1 tablespoon barley malt syrup
1 teaspoon light tahini
1 cup apple juice
3/4 cup roasted ground almonds or pecan nuts
1 1/2 teaspoons agar-agar flakes

1. Slice apples and place in water with salt and raisins. Bring to a boil and simmer for 10 minutes, or until soft.

2. Add barley malt syrup, tahini, apple juice, and nuts to apples and mix well or blend if preferred. Return to the pan.

3. Add agar-agar flakes and stir over heat. Bring to a boil and turn off heat.

4. Allow to set. Refrigerate and serve.

193. Apple-Mango Kanten

Serves 4

2 medium apples
1 cup water
1 cup apple juice
Pinch of salt
1 teaspoon agar-agar
1 mango, sliced
4 fresh mint leaves or cherries

1. Peel and slice the apples. If organic, grate the peel.

2. Bring water and apple juice to a boil and add salt, apples, and grated peel. Lower heat and simmer for 10 minutes.

3. Slice fresh mango into heatproof dish.

4. Strain off stewed apples, reserving the juice, and arrange in dish with mango pieces.

5. Add agar-agar to the juice and stir well over heat. Bring almost to a boil and then turn off heat. Pour juice over the apple, and mango.

6. Leave until set. Place in separate containers if preferred. Refrigerate for 30 minutes.

7. Decorate with a mint leaf, cherry, or dollop of Tofu Cream Whip or Tofutti Cream (*see* Recipes 220 and 222).

194. Apple Pie Filling

8 apples, peeled and sliced
3/4 cup apple juice
1/2 cup raisins
1/2 teaspoon cinnamon

1/4 teaspoon nutmeg
1/2 teaspoon vanilla extract
1 teaspoon agar-agar flakes
2 teaspoons kuzu

1. Preheat oven to 350°F/180°C.

2. Bring 1/2 cup apple juice to a boil with raisins and spices. Boil for half a minute. Sprinkle in agar-agar flakes and stir.

3. Dissolve kuzu in 1/4 cup apple juice, add to the mixture and stir until it begins to boil. Remove from heat.

4. Roll out pastry (*see* Recipes 76, 77, and 78). Place half on the bottom of pie dish.

5. Add apples, pour over the spice sauce and cover with pastry. Decorate and pierce pie crust and place in 400°F/200°C oven for 15 minutes, then 350°F/180°C oven for 30 more minutes.

195. Apple-Tahini Pancake Filling

Serves 4

2 sweet apples, peeled, cored, and sliced
Pinch of salt (optional)
Pinch of cinnamon
1/2 cup raisins
1/2 cup apple juice
2 teaspoons light tahini
1 teaspoon barley malt syrup
1/2 teaspoon kuzu
1/2 cup water (more or less)

1. Cook apples, salt, cinnamon, and raisins in apple juice for 10 minutes.

2. In another pan mix tahini and barley malt syrup. Heat gently until tahini bubbles.

3. Mix kuzu in water and add to the tahini. Stir carefully until mixture is a creamy spread. Add a little more water if necessary.

4. Spread tahini mix then apples over Buckwheat Pancakes (*see* Recipe 74) and fold pancakes over it.

196. Apricot Kanten

Serves 4

1 cup hunza or diced apricots (pitted)
Pinch of salt
3 cups water
Juice of 1 orange
1 1/2 teaspoons agar-agar flakes
1/2 cup roasted almonds or hazelnuts

1. Soak apricots 1 hour. Bring to a boil in water and salt. Sprinkle in agar-agar flakes, simmer and stir. Add orange juice. Allow mixture to cool for 20 minutes.

4. Wet shallow heatproof dish or mold or individual containers. Pour into containers and leave for 30 minutes to set. Refrigerate for another 30 minutes.

5. Decorate with grated almonds or hazelnuts or Tofutti Cream (*see* Recipe 222).

197. Aduki and Raisin Kanten

Serves 4 to 6

1/2 cup aduki beans
1/2 cup raisins
1 strip kombu, 2" x 2"
3 cups water
3 teaspoons agar-agar flakes
3 cups apple juice
1 cup water
1/2 teaspoon vanilla extract

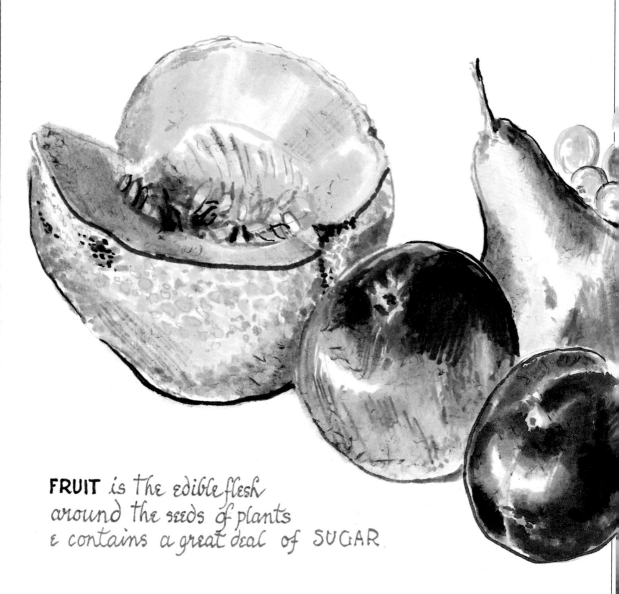

FRUIT is the edible flesh around the seeds of plants & contains a great deal of SUGAR

1. Soak aduki for at least 2 hours, or, if possible, overnight. Discard water.
2. Place aduki beans, raisins, kombu, and water in a pan. Bring to a boil and cook 10 minutes (remember, aduki will swell 5 times or more in volume).
3. Simmer gently for 1 1/2 to 2 hours, or until beans are soft. Add more water if necessary. Let most of it evaporate during the last 1/2 hour of stewing.
4. In another pan heat the apple juice and water with vanilla. Sprinkle agar-agar flakes into it and stir.
5. Add the aduki and raisins. Stir well.
6. Allow to cool; place into containers or mold and let set. Refrigerate for 30 minutes.
7. Decorate with Tofutti Cream (*see* Recipe 222) and a piece of fruit.

Aduki and raisins can be used as a side vegetable dish, for salad, or can be added to rice croquettes.

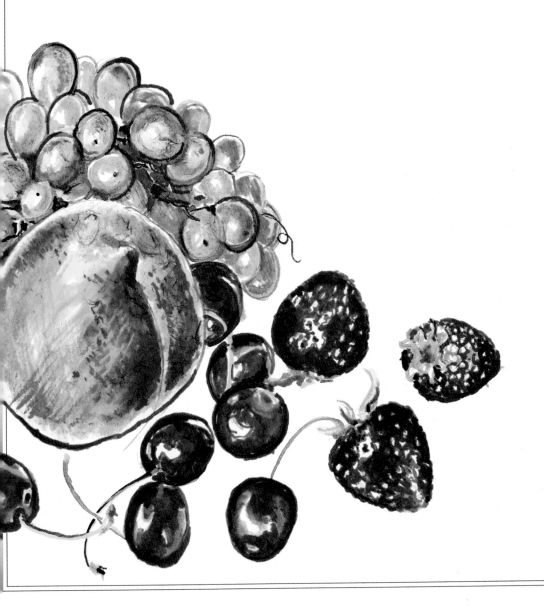

198. Blackberry Kuzu Dessert

Serves 2 to 4

> 1 cup oat milk
> 1 cup apple juice
> 1/4 cup raisins
> 1 tablespoon rice or corn syrup
> 1/2 apple, peeled and sliced
> 2 heaping teaspoons kuzu
> 2 heaping teaspoons fine oatmeal
> 2 heaping teaspoons rice flour
> 2 teaspoons corn flour
> 1/2 cup cold apple juice
> 1 cup blackberries

1. Heat the milk; gently stir in apple juice, raisins, apples, and rice or corn syrup in a pan.

2. Add oatmeal, rice, and corn flour mixed in 1/2 cup apple juice. Simmer over low heat for 5 minutes.

3. Stir kuzu in cup of apple juice, add to first mixture and stir well until mixture thickens and is about to boil.

4. Wash blackberries. Save 6 for garnish and place the remainder in a bowl or separate dessert dishes. Pour mixture over them and allow to cool.

5. Garnish with rest of fruit. Serve with Tofutti Cream (*see* Recipe 222).

Can be made with any fruit in season.

199. Brown Rice Pudding 1

Serves 4

> 1/2 cup apple juice
> 2 cups oat milk
> 1 cup cooked brown rice (*see* INGREDIENTS—Grains)
> 2 teaspoons raisins
> 1/2 teaspoon cinnamon (optional)
> 1 teaspoon rice syrup

1. Preheat oven to 300° F/150° C.

2. Mix oat milk with apple juice in an ovenproof dish.

3. Add rice, raisins, and cinnamon.

4. Bake in preheated oven for 3 hours.

This pudding is delicious when eaten cold.

200. Baked Apples with Tahini Raisins and Lemon (or Orange) Filling

Serves 4

> 4 apples
> 1 1/2 tablespoons tahini
> 1/2 cup raisins
> 2 teaspoons grated, fresh lemon (or orange) peel or marmalade (*see Recipe 217*)
> 1/2 teaspoon cinnamon
> 1 tablespoon grated, roasted walnuts or hazelnuts
> Juice of 1/2 lemon (or orange)
> 4 teaspoons barley malt syrup

1. Preheat oven to 350°F/180°C.
2. Cut a 1" cone shape deep out of the top and bottom of the apple. Remove core of the apple with a knife, leaving a round hollow right through the apple.
3. Mix tahini, raisins, lemon (or orange) peel (or marmalade), cinnamon, and grated walnuts with lemon (or orange) juice and 1 teaspoon of the barley malt syrup.
4. Stuff apples with the mixture. Replace cone in base. This is to prevent the filling from running out while cooking. Gently pierce skin of each apple with a fork.
5. Cook in oven for 15 minutes, or until tender. Remove from oven and pour a little barley malt syrup over each apple. Return to oven for another 5 minutes and then serve.

201. Barley Malt and Kuzu Cream

Serves 4

> 1 cup oat milk
> 2 tablespoons barley malt syrup
> 1 dessertspoon kuzu
> 2 cups apple juice
> 1/2 satsuma or tangerine
> 1/2 cup chopped, toasted hazelnuts or almonds

1. Heat oat milk and add the barley malt syrup, stirring well.
2. Mix kuzu and apple juice and add to the milk, continuing to stir. Bring almost to a boil.
3. Pour into bowls and leave to set 30 to 45 minutes.
4. Break the satsuma into small sections and place one on top of each portion. Sprinkle with chopped, roasted hazelnuts or almonds.

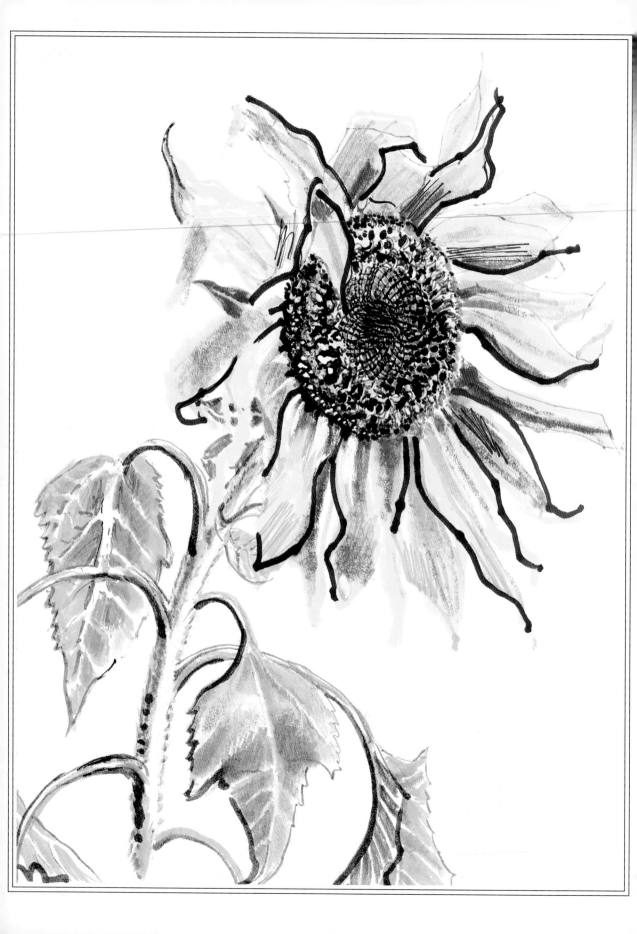

202. Boil and Bake Fruit Cake

One 9" x 9" cake

> 3 cups mixed fruit (seedless raisins, currants, dates, apricots, etc.)
> Peel of 1/2 lemon, grated
> Peel of 1/2 orange, grated
> 1/2 apple, diced
> 1/2 cup mixed nuts, crushed
> 1/2 cup sunflower seeds
> 2 cups apple juice
> 1 cup bancha tea
> 1/3 cup sunflower or sesame oil
> 1 teaspoon cinnamon
> Pinch of salt
> 2 teaspoons fresh, grated ginger
> 2 cups flour
> 1 egg or 1 tablespoon of kuzu mixed in 1 cup apple juice
> 2 teaspoons sesame oil
> 1/4 cup whole wheat flour
> 1 dozen peeled almonds

1. Mix the fruit, nuts, seeds, apple juice, bancha tea, oil, cinnamon, salt, and ginger in a pan. Bring to a boil and simmer gently for 5 minutes.

2. Allow to cool (can stand overnight), then add the flour and egg or kuzu and apple juice. Save a tablespoon of kuzu liquid to glaze cake.

3. Preheat oven to 375°F/190°C. Oil and dust with flour a 9 x 9 cake pan.

4. Stir mixture well and pour into prepared pan.

5. To peel almonds more easily, first immerse in boiling water for 10 minutes. Decorate top of cake with them and brush with kuzu–apple juice mixture to smooth and glaze surface.

6. Bake in preheated oven, on low rack, for 1 hour 15 minutes.

203. Carob "Blancmange"

Serves 4

> 1 teaspoon kuzu
> 1 cup apple juice
> 2 cups rice milk
> Pinch of cinnamon
> 1 tablespoon raisins
> 1 teaspoon carob flour
> 1 tablespoon barley malt syrup
> 2 teaspoons agar-agar
> 6 or 8 pitted cherries

1. Dissolve kuzu in cold water until smooth.

2. Place heatproof bowl in boiling water and add soy milk, cinnamon, raisins, carob flour, and kuzu to bowl. Stir gently until hot.

3. Stir in barley malt syrup and kuzu liquid. Sprinkle in agar-agar and stir well.

4. Add raisins and stir until the mixture is smooth and creamy. Remove from heat before it boils. Allow to cool a little.

6. Pour into a wet mold. Leave 45 minutes to set. Turn out and decorate with the cherries.

204. Carob-Rice Pudding with Carob Sauce

Serves 4

> 2 cups cooked rice
> 1/2 cup apple juice
> 3/4 cup organic soy, oat, or rice milk
> 1 tablespoon rice or corn syrup
> 2 teaspoons chopped raisins
> 1 teaspoon tahini
> 1/2 teaspoon vanilla extract
> 1 teaspoon ground cinnamon

1. Preheat oven to 300°F/150°C.
2. Place cooked rice in an ovenproof Pyrex or ceramic dish. Pour in apple juice, milk, rice or corn syrup, chopped raisins, tahini, and vanilla extract.
3. Sprinkle with cinnamon and bake for 2 1/2 hours.

This pudding improves if kept in a cool place overnight.

CAROB SAUCE

> 1 tablespoon carob flour
> 1/2 cup water
> 1 tablespoon grated orange rind
> 2 teaspoons kuzu
> 1/2 cup apple juice
> 2 tablespoons barley malt syrup
> 1/2 cup orange juice
> 1 heaping tablespoon chopped hazelnuts

1. Mix carob flour with water and add grated orange rind (reserve a little for garnish).
2. Bring to a boil and cook for 20 minutes, stirring well.
3. Dissolve kuzu in cold apple juice, add to carob mixture with barley malt syrup and orange juice, simmer and stir until smooth.
4. Pour mixture over the rice pudding and sprinkle with hazelnuts and remaining orange rind.
5. Cool and serve.

This can also be topped with Cashew and Apple Cream (*see* Recipe 205).

205. Cashew and Apple Cream

Topping for 4 to 6

> 4 golden delicious apples
> 1 cup cashew nuts
> 1 teaspoon vanilla extract
> Pinch of salt

1. Peel and slice apples. Mash apples to a purée, but don't add liquid.
2. Pan-roast cashew nuts dry, stirring for 5 to 10 minutes. Add the apples, salt, and vanilla and blend.
3. Use as a dessert topping (*see* Recipe 204).

206. Couscous Cake

One 10" round cake

> 1 cup seedless raisins (or golden seedless raisins)
> Pinch of salt
> 2 cups apple juice
> 3 cups water
> 1 cup couscous
> 2 teaspoons kuzu
> 1/2 cup apple juice
> 2 tablespoons barley malt syrup (or corn or rice syrup)
> 2 teaspoons fresh ginger juice
> Pinch of salt
> 1 teaspoon agar-agar

1. Simmer raisins in salted apple juice and water for 20 minutes.

2. Pour in the couscous. It should be almost covered. Mix.

3. Simmer 5 minutes (pan covered). Turn off heat. Couscous will swell and rise. Let stand 20 minutes.

4. Place couscous and raisins in shallow 10" round dish.

5. In a sauce pan, mix kuzu in 1/2 cup apple juice. Heat gently.

6. Add the barley malt syrup (or corn or rice syrup), ginger, and salt. Bring to a boil. Sprinkle on agar-agar and stir to make a glaze.

7. Pour over couscous and allow to set for 30 minutes.

As an alternative glaze use Apricot Kanten (*see* Recipe 196), or another fruit kanten can be spread over the top of the cake and allowed to set.

207. Fruit Cake

One 9" x 9" cake

> 3 cups whole wheat flour
> 1/2 cup safflower or sunflower oil
> 1 tablespoon crumbled tofu
> 1/2 teaspoon cinnamon or nutmeg
> 1 cup muesli (*see* Recipe 31)
> 1 cup puffed whole wheat (optional)
> 1/2 cup apple juice
> 1 cup bancha tea
> 1 apple, grated
> 1 cup seedless raisins
> 1/2 cup chopped, mixed nuts
> 1 teaspoon sesame paste
> 2 teaspoons grated, fresh lemon rind or orange rind
> 2 teaspoons grated ginger

1. Preheat oven to 350°F/120°C.

2. Mix flour, oil, tofu, cinnamon or nutmeg, muesli, and puffed wheat.

3. Add apple juice, bancha tea, and apple. Mix in raisins, nuts, sesame paste, grated lemon, and ginger. Let stand for half an hour. Mixture should not be too wet.

4. Place mixture in an oiled 9" x 9" cake pan and bake in preheated oven, on low rack, for 1 hour.

208. Fruit Compote

Serves 4 to 6

>1 Red Delicious (sweet) apple
>1 Golden Delicious (sweet) apple
>1 Granny Smith (tart) apple
>2 ripe pears
>3 dried apricots
>1/4 cup seedless raisins
>1/4 cup apple juice
>1 teaspoon pure vanilla extract

1. Peel, core, and slice apples and pears and place in pot.

2. Slice apricots and add to apples and pears with raisins and apple juice.

3. Bring to a boil and simmer 10 minutes.

4. Add vanilla extract. Serve with muesli or topped with Tofu Cream Whip (*see* Recipe 220).

209. Lemon and Apricot Kanten with Almond Cream

Serves 4

>4 cups apple juice
>1 cup seedless raisins
>1 cup sliced, dry (hunza) apricots
>Juice of 1 lemon, and rind, grated
>Pinch of salt
>2 teaspoons agar-agar flakes

1. Heat apple juice and add raisins, apricots, and lemon rind. Simmer for 1/2 hour. Add salt.

2. Sprinkle in agar-agar and lemon juice and stir into mixture. Bring to a boil and turn off heat. Allow to cool.

3. Pour into individual dishes or a mold. Leave 45 minutes in cool place to set.

4. Top with Almond Cream (*see* Recipe 183), decorate with fresh fruit, and serve.

210. Oatcakes with Raisins

Makes 6

> 1 cup whole wheat pastry flour
> 1 cup oat flakes or muesli (*see Recipe 31*)
> 1 teaspoon cinnamon
> 1/2 cup seedless raisins
> 3 tablespoons oil
> Pinch of salt
> 2 tablespoons oat or barley malt syrup
> 3/4 cup oat milk (more or less)

1. Preheat oven to 450°F/230°C.

2. Mix the ingredients to make a soft dough. Use a little more milk if mixture is too dry.

3. Wet hands and shape into small cakes.

3. Brush oil on baking tray. Sprinkle with a little flour and place cakes on it. Flatten slightly.

4. Bake immediately in preheated oven, on low rack, for 1/2 hour or until golden brown.

Cakes can be rolled in sesame seeds before baking.

211. Oatmeal, Raisin, and Walnut Cookies

Makes 6 to 8

> 1 cup walnuts
> 3/4 cup sunflower seeds
> 1 1/2 cups oats
> 2 tablespoons seedless raisins
> 1 cup apple juice
> 4 teaspoons oat or barley malt syrup
> 1/4 cup mixed sesame and corn oil
> 1/4 teaspoon salt
> 1/2 teaspoon vanilla extract
> 3/4 cup rice flour
> 1 cup rye flour
> 1/2 teaspoon baking powder

1. Preheat oven to 300°F/150°C.

2. Pan-roast walnuts and sunflower seeds, stirring for 5 minutes, and then blend or crush.

3. Soak oats in apple juice for 1/2 hour.

4. Mix syrup with raisins, oil, salt, and vanilla.

5. Mix rice flour, rye flour, and baking powder.

6. Combine all ingredients, add nuts, and stir well.

7. Place cookies on an oiled baking sheet and bake on middle rack in a 300°F oven for 30 to 40 minutes, or until golden brown. Do not overcook.

212. Oatcakes with Pear and Apple Spread

Makes about 12

Dry ingredients:

>2 cups oat flakes or 2 cups muesli (*see* Recipe 31)
>1/2 cup whole wheat flour
>1/2 cup chopped seedless raisins
>1/4 cup chopped hazelnuts
>1/4 cup chopped almonds

Wet ingredients:

>3 tablespoons sunflower oil
>1 tablespoon barley malt syrup
>2 tablespoons sunflower butter (or tahini)
>1 tablespoon oat milk
>2 tablespoons pear and apple spread or whole fruit jam (no sugar)

Decoration:

>12 almonds
>1 cup boiling water

1. Preheat oven to 300°F/150°C.

2. Mix dry ingredients.

3. Gently heat and stir with a wooden spoon, syrup, oil, and sunflower butter (or tahini). Pour over dry ingredients.

4. Mix thoroughly. Add milk to make a firm doughy mixture.

5. Form mixture into golf ball shapes, press them flat, and place them on an oiled baking sheet.

6. Make an indentation in the top of each cookie and fill with a little pear and apple spread.

7. Bake in preheated oven, on low rack, for 20 minutes.

8. Soak almonds in boiling water for 10 minutes to remove the skins. Press an almond on top of each cookie. Bake another 15 minutes at 325°F/160°C or until golden brown.

213. Pears Belle Hélène

Serves 4

>4 pears (peeled)
>2 cups water
>Pinch of salt
>1 cup seedless raisins
>1 cup water
>Pinch of salt
>3/4 cup grain or barley coffee or dandelion root coffee
>3 cups water
>1 cup freshly oven-roasted hazelnuts
>2 teaspoons kuzu
>1/2 cup water

1. Immerse pears in boiling water. Add pinch of salt. Simmer gently for 15 minutes, or until soft.

2. Remove pears (discard water) and place them in separate dessert dishes.

3. Soak the raisins for 1/2 hour or longer. Boil in water and salt for 10 minutes.

4. Make the grain or dandelion root coffee—a thick brew—and strain; then add to the raisins.

5. Blend or chop the hazelnuts fine. Add to the mixture.

6. Mix kuzu in water. Add to the sauce and bring to a boil to thicken.

7. Serve on top of pears.

214. Pecan Cream

Topping for 4

>1 cup pecans
>1 cup oat milk
>2 teaspoons barley malt syrup
>1/2 teaspoon vanilla extract
>1/2 teaspoon agar-agar powder

1. Roast nuts gently in a pan until fragrant.

2. Heat milk, stir in barley malt syrup and pour over the pecans.

3. Purée mixture in blender with vanilla and agar-agar powder.

4. Bring to a boil, allow to cool, and refrigerate overnight. Blend again. This should be a light, creamy texture and not too thick. If too thick, add a little water.

5. Use as a dessert topping.

215. Pumpkin or Squash Pie

Makes 1 8" pie

>3 pounds pumpkin or squash, peeled and diced
>3 cups water
>1 tablespoon raisins
>1 teaspoon cinnamon
>1/4 teaspoon nutmeg
>2 teaspoons barley or corn malt syrup
>1 teaspoon vanilla extract
>2 free-range eggs or 2 teaspoons agar-agar flakes
>1 1/2 teaspoons kuzu

1. Place pumpkin or squash in pan with water, bring to a boil, and simmer for 45 minutes, or until soft.

2. Blend pumpkin and remaining water to a smooth cream and return to pan.

3. Add raisins, cinnamon, nutmeg, syrup, and vanilla.

4. If not using eggs, mix kuzu in 1/2 cup cold water and add to mixture. Sprinkle on agar-agar flakes and stir until almost to a boil. Remove from heat. Let cool for 1/2 hour. Alternatively, beat eggs until fluffy and pour into mixture. Stir in thoroughly.

5. Preheat oven to 450°F/230°C.

6. Press out pastry crust into an 8" pie pan (*see* Recipes 76 and 77) and pour mixture into shell, allowing 1/4" for rising.

7. Bake in preheated oven for 10 minutes, then in a 350°F/180°C oven for 30 minutes. The pie is done when a knife blade inserted near the center comes out clean.

216. Rolled Oats and Rolled Barley Cookies

Makes 24 bar cookies

>3/4 cup rolled oats
>3/4 cup roasted wheat flakes or puffed whole wheat
>3/4 cup rolled barley
>1/2 cup chopped, mixed nuts
>1/2 cup raisins
>3 teaspoons safflower oil
>2 tablespoons barley malt syrup
>1 tablespoon rice syrup
>1 cup pastry dough (see Recipe 77)

1. Preheat oven to 400°F/200°C.
2. Mix oats, wheat flakes, barley, nuts, and raisins.
3. Melt barley malt and rice syrup and mix with the oil over low heat.
4. Pour syrups and oil into dry ingredients and stir together.
5. Press pastry thinly into a 9" x 12" baking pan.
6. Press mixture firmly onto pastry. Mark out 24 squares with knife.
7. Bake in middle of preheated oven for 20 minutes, or until golden brown.
8. Remove from tray and cut or break into the squares.

217. Sugarless Compotes

A "sugarless" compote can be made by cooking unpeeled, sliced, and cored apples for 1/2 hour to 45 minutes with half their measure of grape juice or apple juice until 1/4 of the volume of liquid remains. This can be strained if a clear jam is required or left as it is. Fruit is then added and the further cooking time depends on the fruit. Whole strawberries require 5 minutes, apples or pears (sliced) 15 minutes, apricots (pitted, sliced) 15 minutes, cherries (pitted) 20 minutes, oranges 45 minutes (see below).

SWEET ORANGE MARMALADE

Makes 2 to 3 8-ounce jars

>4 sweet oranges
>4 cups pure, unsugared grape or apple juice
>2 organic apples, unpeeled, cored and diced
>1/2 teaspoon salt
>18" square piece of muslin or cheesecloth

1. Scrub oranges gently and wipe. Cut each in half and extract juice.
2. Add juice to grape or apple juice.
3. Remove seeds and pith from oranges and tie securely in the muslin.
4. Place this with fruit juices and apple in pan and bring to a boil. Simmer for 45 minutes or until 1/3 of the liquid remains. Strain if clear jam is required. Add salt.
5. Slice orange skin fine or thick according to preference, add to the juice and boil for 30 to 45 minutes. Squeeze out muslin bag and remove. Marmalade is ready when a drop of the liquid sets on a cold plate.
6. Place canning jars and lids in a 212°F/100°C oven for 20 minutes to sterilize. Ladle the jam into each jar and seal with a lid. Allow to cool, then store. Once opened the jam must be refrigerated.

218. Tahini and Apple Custard

Serves 4

> 1/2 cup raisins
> 2 1/2 cups apple juice
> 3 apples peeled and sliced
> 2 tablespoons tahini
> Pinch of salt
> Pinch of fresh-grated lemon peel
> 4 teaspoons agar-agar flakes
> 1/2 cup grated, roasted almonds.

1. Soak raisins in apple juice for 1 hour or so, then bring to a boil and simmer for 5 minutes.
2. Add the sliced apples. Bring to a boil. Reserve some of the apple for decoration.
3. Add tahini, salt, and grated lemon peel. Sprinkle agar-agar flakes over and stir well.
4. Remove from heat and allow to set for 30 minutes.
5. Blend mixture. Refrigerate for 20 minutes. Serve cold in separate bowls. Decorate with apple slices and sprinkle grated almonds on top.

219. Tarte Tatin (Sweet or Savory)

Serves 4 to 6

> 1/2 cup cornmeal
> 1/2 cup oat flour
> 1/2 cup plain whole wheat flour
> 2 ounces vegetable margarine
> 1/2 cup cold water
> 2 fresh apples (or pears, apricots, or other fruit in season)
> 1 teaspoon raisins
> 4 soft dried apricots (not for apricot Tatin)
> 1/4 teaspoon cinnamon
> 1 teaspoon corn or rice syrup
> zest of orange peel
> Juice of 1/2 an orange
> 1 pinch of sea salt

1. Preheat oven to 400°F/200°C.
2. Mix the flours and sprinkle in salt. Rub the margarine in until mixture is crumbly.
3. Add water, gradually kneading the dough until it is soft.
4. On the bottom of a shallow, 8" ovenproof dish, arrange dried apricots. Peel, core, and slice apples (or other seasonal fruit) and arrange on top of the apricots. Mix syrup, orange juice, orange zest, and salt and pour over apples. Sprinkle with cinnamon.
5. Roll out pastry and place on top of the fruit. Tuck in to cover fruit, but do not seal edges.
6. Bake in preheated oven for 30 minutes. To serve, invert a plate over the tart and turn the tart upside down onto the plate. Serve fruit side up, perhaps with custard (*see Recipe 224*).

SAVORY ONION TATIN

A savory onion Tatin can be made by slicing 3 medium onions lengthwise into large wedges, arrange in an 8" baking dish. Drizzle with a tablespoon of oil, and sprinkle with a teaspoon of fresh thyme. Bake in 400°F/180°C oven for 20 minutes. Pour 2 teaspoons umeboshi vinegar and 2 teaspoons barley or rice malt syrup over onions. Cover with pastry, tuck in but don't seal. When rolling out pastry, sprinkle on 2 teaspoons of grated Peccorino cheese, fold, and roll. Bake another 1/2 hour. Invert to serve.

220. Tofu Cream Whip

Serves 4

> 2 cups diced tofu
> 2 teaspoons vanilla extract
> 1 tablespoon corn syrup
> 1 teaspoon dandelion or grain coffee
> 1 teaspoon tahini
> 1/2 cup apple juice
> 1/2 cup rice milk

1. Blend tofu with vanilla, syrup, coffee, and tahini.

2. Add apple juice and milk to mixture while blending. Take care or the whip may become liquid.

3. Serve as a topping for kantens or pies.

221. Tofu, Rice, and Apricot Whip

Serves 4

> 1 cup hunza dried apricots (if available), pitted
> 3 cups water
> 1 teaspoon kuzu
> 1 teaspoon corn flour
> 2 cups well-cooked, soft whole grain rice (*see* INGREDIENTS—Grains)
> 2 teaspoons barley malt syrup
> 1 cup diced tofu
> 1 cup apple juice
> 1/2 teaspoon cinnamon
> 1/2 cup roasted pecan nuts

1. Soak apricots for 1 hour and boil until soft (1/2 hour) and most of the liquid has evaporated.

2. Mix kuzu and corn flour well in apple juice, add apricots, and bring almost to a boil.

3. Blend the rice, barley malt syrup, tofu, and cinnamon. Place in a bowl and stir in apricots.

4. Decorate with chopped pecan nuts.

222. Tofutti Cream

Topping for 4

> 1/2 cup apple juice
> 2 fresh apples, diced

2 teaspoons barley malt syrup
2 teaspoons kuzu
1/2 cup cold apple juice
1/2 cup roasted hazelnuts
3 cups diced tofu
1/2 teaspoon vanilla extract

1. Heat apple juice in pan. Add apples and barley malt syrup. Bring to a boil.

2. Add kuzu in cold apple juice to fruit. Stir until mixture thickens. Remove from heat just before boiling. Allow to cool.

3. Blend the nuts and add the fruit mixture, tofu, and vanilla. Blend to make a cream.

4. Refrigerate and use to decorate sweet dishes.

One and one half cups of fruit in season—strawberries, blackberries, cherries, pears, grapes—can be used instead of apple.

223. Tofu and Walnut Pie

Serves 4 to 6

1 cup ground, roasted walnuts or hazelnuts
2 cups tofu, crumbled
1/2 cup water
1/2 cup oat milk
2 teaspoons barley malt, rice, or corn syrup
1/2 teaspoon vanilla extract
1 cup apple juice
1 teaspoon agar-agar flakes

1. Blend walnuts (or hazelnuts) and add tofu, water, oat milk, barley malt syrup and vanilla extract. Blend these ingredients.

2. Heat apple juice in pan and sprinkle on agar-agar flakes. Stir until dissolved. Bring to a boil and then turn off heat.

3. Add the walnut mixture and stir well.

4. Pour into a cooked pastry crust (*see* Recipes 76, 77, 78, 81). Allow to cool and then refrigerate for 30 minutes before serving.

224. Vanilla Custard 1

Serves 4

2 cups soy or rice milk
1/2 teaspoon seeds scraped from a vanilla pod
1 tablespoon raisins
2 teaspoons rice syrup or barley malt syrup
Pinch of ground turmeric for color (optional)
2 teaspoons kuzu

1. Place 1 1/2 cups soy milk and the vanilla in a pan with raisins, rice syrup, and turmeric (if yellow color is desired). Heat and stir.

2. Mix the kuzu in 1/2 cup cold soy milk and add to the pan. Stir well, until the custard thickens.

3. Serve over sweet dishes, hot or cold.

225. Vanilla Custard 2

Serves 4

> 1 cup organic soy, rice, or oat milk
> 1/2 teaspoon vanilla extract or seeds scraped from a vanilla pod
> Pinch of ground turmeric or 2 to 3 threads of saffron (to color—optional)
> 1 tablespoon corn syrup
> 2 teaspoons agar-agar flakes
> 2 teaspoons kuzu
> 2 teaspoons cornmeal
> 1 teaspoon finely ground oatmeal (oat flour)
> 1/2 cup additional soy, rice, or oat milk

1. Heat 1 cup of the milk, vanilla, and turmeric or saffron. Add syrup and agar-agar. Bring to a boil.

2. Mix kuzu, cornmeal and oatmeal in 1/2 cup soy, rice, or oat milk. Pour into custard and stir.

3. Bring to a boil and then remove from heat. Allow to cool and set or serve hot over sweet dishes.

226. Walnut or Pecan Cookies

Makes 9 to 12 cookies

> 2 cups whole wheat pastry flour
> 2 tablespoons corn oil
> 1 cup ground, roasted walnuts or pecans
> 1 free-range egg
> 1 tablespoon barley malt or rice syrup
> 1 teaspoon cinnamon
> 1/4 teaspoon vanilla extract

1. Preheat oven to 375°F/200°C.

2. Mix ingredients to make a soft biscuit dough.

3. Brush cookie sheet with oil and dust with flour. Spoon dough onto sheet. Flatten slightly.

4. Bake on middle rack of preheated oven for 1/2 hour.

227. Wheat Flake and Malt Cookies

Makes 6 to 8 cookies

> 1/2 cup sesame oil
> 1 tablespoon barley malt syrup
> 1 tablespoon tofu
> 1 teaspoon vanilla extract
> 1 tablespoon oat milk or organic soy milk
> 1 cup whole wheat flour
> 1/2 teaspoon salt
> 2 cups whole wheat flakes or puffed whole wheat
> 1/2 cup chopped raisins
> 1/4 cup shredded coconut
> 1 teaspoon grated lemon rind
> 1/4 cup water

1. Preheat oven to 350°F/180°C.

2. Mix first 5 ingredients. Stir in remaining ingredients. Add a few drops of water if needed.

3. Using a teaspoon, drop 2" apart onto an oiled cookie sheet and bake on middle rack of oven for 30 minutes.

Some Suggested Menus

Spring Menus

I.

BREAKFAST:
- Shiro miso soup (*see* Recipe 14) or
  Boiled brown rice or noodles in miso soup
- Bannocks (*see* Recipe 69) with hummus (*see* Recipe 141), pressed salad (*see* Recipe 117), and nori spread (*see* Recipe 149) or with tahini and sweet orange marmalade (*see* Recipe 217)
- Kukicha (twig) tea (*see* INGREDIENTS—Kukicha)

LUNCH:
- Udon brown rice/noodles with tofu "Alfredo" sauce (*see* Recipe 63) and water sautéed cabbage (see Recipe 104 for procedure)
- Slice of fruit cake (*see* Recipe 207) or
  Apricot Kanten (*see* Recipe 196)
- Green tea or
  Apple juice

DINNER:
- Sushi (*see* Recipe 124)
- Pancakes (see Recipe 80) with béchamel vegetable sauce (see Recipe 111)
- Kombu and carrots (*see* Recipe 106) or
  Aduki and parsnip (*see* Recipe 129; substitute parsnip for pumpkin) or
  Cabbage and caraway-tofu sauce (*see* Recipe 139) or
  Spring greens, water sautéed (*see* Recipe 104 for procedure)
- Millet and cauliflower mash (*see* Recipe 51) or
  Boiled brown rice (*see* INGREDIENTS—Rice)
- Daikon and umeboshi vinegar (*see* Recipe 99)
- Couscous cake (*see* Recipe 206) or
  Carob and rice pudding with carob sauce (*see* Recipe 205)
- Barley tea (mugicha)

2.

BREAKFAST:

- Pinhead oat porridge (*see* INGREDIENTS—Grains) served with stewed apricots and rice syrup (1 teaspoon) with rice or oat milk
- Whole wheat bread (*see* Recipe 83) or bannocks (*see* Recipe 69) served with
  Hummus (see Recipe 141) or nori spread (*see* Recipe 149) or
  Tahini and ginger spread (*see* Recipe 156) or sugar-free orange marmalade (*see* Recipe 217)

LUNCH:

- Guacamole and corn chips (*see* Recipe 142)
- Millet and baked parsnips with vegetables (*see* Recipe 53) with pressed salad (*see* Recipe 117)
- Tofu cheese with crackers or bannocks
- Bancha tea

DINNER:

- Onion and dulse soup (*see* Recipe 21) with tamari
- Tempuraed vegetables, tofu, and prawns (optional) (*see* INGREDIENTS—Tempura and Recipe 113) with boiled brown rice (*see* INGREDIENTS—Rice)
- Chinese pressed cabbage (*see* Recipe 97, 98) or
  Sliced dill cucumber pickles (*see* Recipe 114)
- Pears Belle Hélène (*see* Recipe 213)
- Roasted grain coffee

Summer Menus

I.

BREAKFAST:

- Breakfast muesli (*see* Recipe 31) soaked in apple juice (1/2 hour) with oat milk and stewed apples and raisins
- Corn, rye, and whole wheat bread (*see* Recipe 71) with
  tahini, ginger, and scallion miso spread (*see* Recipe 156) or
  Sweet orange marmalade (*see* Recipe 217)
- Kukicha (twig) tea

LUNCH:

- Rice, avocado, and corn salad (*see* Recipe 58) with
  aduki beans (*see* INGREDIENTS—Legumes) and broccoli with
  roasted pumpkin seeds (*see* Recipe 88)
- Wheat flake and malt cookies (*see* Recipe 227) or
  Tofu and walnut pie (*see* Recipe 223)
- Hojicha or bancha tea

DINNER:

- Crab and sweet corn soup (*see* Recipe 169)
- Sweet boiled carrots (*see* Recipe 125) with a dip of hummus (*see* Recipe 141)
- Polenta patties with vegetables (*see* Recipe 57) with water-sautéed kale (*see* Recipe 104) or Mustard greens with pumpkin seed salad (*see* Recipe 109)
- Tofu and walnut pie (*see* Recipe 223) with vanilla custard (*see* Recipes 224 and 225) or Amazake and pear "blancmange" (*see* Recipe 185)
- Dandelion or grain coffee

2.

BREAKFAST:

- Cold whole oat or pinhead porridge (*see* INGREDIENTS—Grains) blended with some stewed apple and raisin and decorated with fresh or cooked fruit in season (grated apple, sliced peach, pitted cherries, or strawberries) with a sprinkling of rice, oat, or barley malt syrup and rice or oat milk
- Bannocks (*see* Recipe 69) or toasted whole wheat bread (*see* Recipe 83) with hummus (*see* Recipe 141), or nori spread (*see* Recipe 149), and pressed salad (*see* Recipe 117) or apple and pear spread (*see* Recipe 217)
- Kukicha (twig) tea or/bancha tea

LUNCH:

- Brown rice summer salad (*see* Recipe 38)
- Oatcake or sourdough and onion bread (*see* Recipe 73) with tofu-dill salad spread (*see* Recipe 161)
- Sauerkraut (*see* Recipe 115)
- Apricot kanten (*see* Recipe 196)
- Genmaicha (*see* INGREDIENTS—Green Tea) or apple juice

DINNER:

- Guacamole (*see* Recipe 142) served with
  corn, rye, and whole wheat bread (*see* Recipe 71) or
  corn chips (unsalted or with sea salt or tamari flavor)
- Couscous (*see* Recipe 44) served with
  aduki and summer squash (*see* Recipe 129; substitute summer squash for pumpkin)
- Carrot, dulse, and celery boiled salad (*see* Recipe 91) or
  Watercress and orange salad (*see* Recipe 128)
- Carob "blancmange" (*see* Recipe 204)
- Mint tea with fresh mint

Autumn Menus

I.

BREAKFAST:

- Whole oat porridge (*see* Recipe 32) served with
  blackberries and apples stewed with raisins and a teaspoon of corn and barley malt syrup
  with a dash of organic soy milk
- Whole grain bread (*see* Recipes 71 and 72) with
  tofu cheese (*see* Recipe 160) and/or nori spread (*see* Recipe 149)
- Mugicha (*see* INGREDIENTS—Barley)

LUNCH:

- Pumpkin and miso soup (*see* Recipe 23) with the addition of some boiled, whole grain rice
  sprinkled with gomasio and/or shiso condiment (*see* INGREDIENTS—Gomasio and Shiso)
- Oatcakes with raisins (*see* Recipe 210) or
  Oatmeal raisin and walnut cookies (*see* Recipe 211)
- Kukicha (twig) tea or bancha tea

DINNER:

- Lentil pâté (*see* Recipe 107) served with corn and rye bread (*see* Recipe 71) or
  Rolled oats and celery soup (*see* Recipe 24) with wholegrain bread croûtons
- Udon brown rice noodles (*see* INGREDIENTS—Noodles) with mushroom and red pepper
  sea salad sauce (*see* Recipe 66) and
  Broccoli with roasted pumpkin seeds (*see* Recipe 88) or
  Aduki and pumpkin (*see* Recipe 129) and/or
  Carrot, scallion, and snow pea salad (*see* Recipe 92) or snow pea and ginger salad (*see*
  Recipe 108)
- Pumpkin or squash pie (*see* Recipe 215) with pecan cream (*see* Recipe 214) or
  Brown rice pudding (*see* Recipe 199)
- Mu tea with a dash of apple juice

2.

BREAKFAST:

- Dashi (*see* INGREDIENTS—Dashi) with noodles or
  Whole wheat flakes (unsugared) with compote of stewed apples and raisins with oat milk
- Pan-toasted corn, rye, and whole wheat bread (*see* Recipe 71) with tahini, ginger, and
  scallion miso spread (*see* Recipe 156) or tahini and unsugared jam (*see* Recipe 217)
- Kukicha (twig) tea

LUNCH:

- Rice and bean croquettes (*see* Recipe 59) served hot with mochi and onion sauce (*see* Recipe
  146) with
  Grated carrot, raisin, and lettuce with apple juice and tamari salad dressing (*see* Recipe 153)

- Slice of fruit cake (*see* Recipe 207) or
  Fruit compote (*see* Recipe 208)
- Twig tea

DINNER:

- Cold borscht soup (*see* Recipe 3)
- Paella (*see* Recipe 172) served with
  Broccoli, steamed, with toasted pumpkin seeds (*see* Recipe 88) or
  Radish flowers and umeboshi kanten (*see* Recipe 119) or
  Sauerkraut and radish kanten (*see* Recipe 122) or
  Watercress, orange, and onion salad (*see* Recipe 128)
- Apple and blackberry crumble (*see* Recipe 187) or
  Lemon and apricot kanten (*see* Recipe 209) topped with almond cream (*see* Recipe 183)
- Mu tea and apple juice or
  Roasted grain coffee

Winter Menus

I.

BREAKFAST:

- Whole oat porridge (*see* Recipe 32) with cooked rice blended, topped with a teaspoonful of
  pressed carrot, daikon, and cucumber salad (*see* Recipe 117), and served with sesame salt,
  tamari, and a dash of oat milk
- Bannocks (*see* Recipe 69) with pressed salad (*see* Recipe 117), tahini (*see* INGREDIENTS) or
  hummus (*see* Recipe 141) and nori spread (*see* Recipe 149) or
  Bread of five grains (*see* Recipe 72) with tahini, ginger, and scallion miso spread (*see* Recipe 156)
- Bancha tea or twig tea

LUNCH:

- Miso soup (*see* Recipe 14) with bread (*see* Recipe 70) and tofu-dill salad spread (*see* Recipe 161)
- Oatcakes with raisins (*see* Recipe 210) or
  Slice of boil and bake fruitcake (*see* Recipe 202)
- Bancha tea or Kukicha (twig) tea

DINNER:

- Pumpkin soup (*see* Recipe 22) with Mochi croutons (*see* INGREDIENTS—Mochi) or
  Prawns and sesame toast (*see* Recipe 174)
- Millet-aduki croquettes (*see* Recipe 49) with béchamel cheese sauce (*see* Recipe 137) or with
  onion and squash sauce (*see* Recipe 151) with
  Steamed broccoli (*see* Recipe 88) with roasted pumpkin seeds or
  Sweet boiled carrots (*see* Recipe 125) or
  Hijiki with onion, carrots, and nuts (*see* Recipe 101) or
  Carrot and turnip cooked salad (*see* Recipe 93)
- Tarte tatin (*see* Recipe 219) or
  Tahini and apple custard (*see* Recipe 218)
- Mugicha (*see* INGREDIENTS—Barley)

2.

BREAKFAST:

- Miso, dulse, and onion soup with tofu (*see* Recipe 15) with
  cooked noodles added or
  Whole oat porridge (*see* Recipe 32) served with 1 teaspoon of sauerkraut (*see* Recipe 115) or
  a small sliced dill cucumber pickle (*see* Recipe 114) or
  tamari and shiso condiment (*see* INGREDIENTS—Shiso) and oat milk
- Bannocks (*see* Recipe 69) or
  Bread (*see* Recipe 70) with tahini, ginger, and scallion miso spread (*see* Recipe 156) or
  apple and pear spread (available commercially with no sugar added; *see also* Recipe 217)
- Bancha tea or Kukicha (twig) tea or
  Roasted grain coffee

LUNCH:

- Brown rice, aduki beans, and vegetables (*see* Recipe 33) with sesame salt and tamari
- Slice of boil and bake fruit cake (*see* Recipe 202)
- Genmaicha (*see* INGREDIENTS—Green Tea)

DINNER:

- Watercress soup (*see* Recipe 28)
- Tempeh and mochi layers stew (*see* Recipe 133) or
  Tempeh with tahini and miso cream sauce (*see* Recipe 134) with boiled rice or millet and
  Steamed brussels sprouts (*see* Recipe 88 for procedure) or
  Kale and mushrooms, boiled (*see* Recipe 103) or
  Kombu and carrots (*see* Recipe 106)
- Dill cucumber pickles (*see* Recipe 114) or
  Cauliflower in umeboshi vinegar (*see* Recipe 95)
- Baked apple (*see* Recipe 200) with vanilla custard (*see* Recipe 224) or
  Apple pie (*see* Recipe 190) with tofuti cream (*see* Recipe 222)
- Dandelion coffee or
  Roasted grain coffee

Any Suggestions?

I suppose I had now better admit that Ohsawa had a poor opinion of actors. They were low in his seven levels of judgment and health, as "sellers of pleasure," and were, in his opinion, "gourmands and greedy." Perhaps he didn't know many actors—or perhaps he did! But suggesting to an actor that he should be in bed, like everyone else, before midnight and should not eat three hours before getting there is rather difficult if the actor has to work in the theater at night! It is, though, generally a sound suggestion and worth remembering.

There is much that is wise in macrobiotics, and the traditional remedies and diagnoses that Ohsawa and Michio Kushi detail in their books are worth reading. They both make wise and practical suggestions for a "harmonious and healthy way of life."

The Unique Principle does provide a compass and a state of mind that is glad for life and natural things. Eating naturally can also help the appreciation of natural fibers in clothing and furnishings. Wearing a fabric such as cotton, for example, next to the skin is pleasanter and healthier than wearing synthetics. Too much metallic jewelry around the neck, wrists, and fingers especially can affect the joints and skin.

Swimming in the ocean with its mineral content is naturally better for you than luxuriating in a chlorinated pool. When bathing or taking a shower use a loofa or brush on your skin and finish with a cold shower unless your doctor says otherwise. Try rubbing yourself down thoroughly with a hot, damp towel each day. This is especially good for the hands, fingers, feet, and toes. Baths can be a relaxing yin treatment after a hard yang day's work, but soaking for hours in hot water is rather like soaking your vegetables for too long—the body can be drained of minerals! Most "bath salts," and even oils, can contain frothy detergents and strong, chemically perfumed cosmetics that not only smell harsh but are tough on the skin.

Take a half hour of fresh-as-possible air each day by walking or gently jogging—on grass if possible or on sand—even in bare feet if it is safe. Most cities have a park where there are trees and grass.

Give plants space in your home. With a liitle care, plants can live with you for years and will become great friends. They look good and help keep the air fresh during the day. The temperature of your rooms needs to be kept as natural as possible, without too much reliance on central heating or air conditioning. Open windows whenever you can, let in air and enjoy the seasons.

Perhaps one of the most important health factors, next to food, is exercise. As "sellers of the physical," actors are probably more aware than most of how necessary it is to keep the body functioning as smoothly as possible. Sitting for long periods while writing this book has made me realize how uncomfortable desk work can be and how vital it is to do some sort of regular exercise. The older one gets the more important it is. Any type of exercise is worthwhile, from yoga to gentle walking, jogging, or lifting light weights. (Many more gyms and health centers have opened all over the world since this book was first written.) Nan Bronfen says, "Exercise helps keep minerals in the bones and strengthens them. Lack of stress or weight-bearing movements causes bone reabsorption. Exercise that delivers rapid impact is more effective in generating the right kind of electrical stimulation. Walking is excellent exercise, and weight-lifting exercises are better than swimming in this respect."

Especially Macrobiotics!

While reading for the next sections on nutrition I came across several warnings concerning macrobiotics, which are well worth mentioning.

Carl C. Pfeiffer, PhD., M.D., in *Mental and Elemental Nutrients*, seems to jump to a common conclusion about Regimen 7—the brown rice only diet. He assumes, as did some others in the early days of macrobiotics, that the aim of all macrobiotics is to pass through the seven stages of eating, I quote Pfeiffer, "reducing the variety of food ingested purportedly to help the individual achieve well-being, spiritual awakening, or rebirth . . . until the last stage when all that one ingests is brown rice and tea." He goes on to stress emphatically, and quite correctly, the dangers of making a habit of the brown rice only diet.

George Ohsawa, who claimed that "the happy man eats anything he wants with great joy and gratitude," was also of the opinion that most sickness was produced by excesses of food. He recommended a diet of brown rice only, which he called Regimen 7, from time to time to recover physically and mentally from the effects of such excesses. "Grain fasts such as Regimen 7 can include small amounts of seasoning, condiments, and liquid, and the *whole* grains can be prepared in various ways—as porridge or gruel, pancakes, bread, noodles, chapatis, etc.," says Michio Kushi, who warns that grain fasts such as Regimen 7 should not last longer than two weeks at a time unless under experienced supervision. To eat nothing but rice for weeks on end is dangerous—and very boring! You may get away with it in a Zen monastery or on top of a mountain but not when living an average life in the middle of any large modern city, with all its strain, stress, and pollution.

If, however, you are not feeling well—usually because of something you have eaten—just one day on brown rice, with a few vegetables and kuzu sauce makes all the difference. Try it!

Another interesting reference to macrobiotics is found in Frances Moore Lappe's excellent book, *Diet for a Small Planet*. A quotation from the *Berkeley Tribe* in 1970 states, "Several cases of severe protein malnutrition (*kwashiorkor*—a disease native to North Africa) have been found in Berkeley. An unpublished University of California hospital report blames certain fasting, vegetarian, and *especially macrobiotic* diets for this. These diets often result in clinically protein-deficient peoples."

Frances Moore Lappe deals with "Complementary Proteins," the combination of nonmeat foods producing high-grade protein equivalent to or even better than meat proteins. The combining of grains and beans, for example, to boost protein has been practiced for centuries by many different civilizations, and mabrobiotics use beans and bean products (tofu, tempeh, tamari, and miso) for cooking. Tempeh also guarantees a supply of Vitamin B$_{12}$ that can be lacking in a completely vegetarian diet.

In California during the sixties there were stories about young people practicing—or malpracticing—macrobiotics. Stories of dehydration, kidney failure, of a young man who drank a whole bottle of soy sauce to yangize himself, of others not drinking enough liquid or eating nothing but rice for weeks on end. Balance is the essence of yin and yang. Common sense tells us that extremes can be dangerous, and we don't have to be philosophers to realize that.

However, in August 1982, *Life* magazine featured an article about a Dr. Anthony Sattilaro, complete with photographs and oscilloscope pictures of his bone scan taken in May 1978. The scan showed dark shadows, cancerous lesions, at the top of his skull, right shoulder, left rib cage, back, and sternum. Soon after this scan was taken Dr. Sattilaro was to lose his father from the same disease. He was, in fact, driving back to Philadelphia from the funeral when he picked up two hitchhikers. Both men were in their early twenties and were macrobiotic students. One of them, Sean McLean, told this doctor who had practiced medicine for twenty years that a change of diet could reverse his condition — that he didn't have to die. "When you eat lots of red meat, dairy products, eggs, refined foods like sugar and white flour, and foods high in preservatives, then you get cancer — if you don't die of a heart attack first!"

"I just looked at him," said Dr. Sattilaro, "and thought he was a silly kid. What could a twenty-five-year-old cook know about cancer?" But in time he chose to think of those two kids as angels. Fourteen months later, after a strict macrobiotic regimen supervised by the Philadelphia East West Foundation, his bone scan showed that Dr. Sattilaro was free of the illness. He admits that one case history is insufficient evidence, but following his recovery he made many innovative changes at the hospital of which he was president and began scientific studies exploring the role of nutrition in cancer and other degenerative diseases.

Ten Regimens to Health and Happiness

To "achieve a state of well being," George Ohsawa recommended using vegetables and grains (instead of animal products) in various proportions. "Regimen 7 is the simplest, the easiest, and wisest," he said. "Try it for 10 days."

DIET #	CEREALS	VEGETABLES	SOUP	ANIMAL	SALADS FRUITS	DESSERT	BEVERAGES
7	100%						Cut down on liquids but don't forget to drink between meals. Bear in mind that soups, boiled or steamed vegetables, and grains contain a high percentage of water. Drink at the end of a meal rather than while eating.
6	90%	10%					
5	80%	20%					
4	70%	20%	10%				
3	60%	30%	10%				
2	50%	30%	10%	10%			
1	40%	30%	10%	20%			
-1	30%	30%	10%	20%	10%		
-2	20%	30%	10%	25%	10%	5%	
-3	10%	30%	10%	30%	15%	5%	

Adapted from George Ohsawa *Zen Macrobiotics.*

The Body — A Laboratory

"We human beings," said Carl C. Pfeiffer, "are biochemicals, if you'll pardon such a pragmatic definition. Everything in the universe is technically a chemical and some of the most beneficial biochemicals, by our standards, are contained in our food, air, and water. These are the nutrients that evolved with life, the vitamins and minerals natural to our food and bodies."

The sun's energy is confined by plants with chemicals such as carbon dioxide, water, nitrogen, and minerals to produce a naturally balanced supply of nutrients for our body's use. You might say we are motivated by solar power!

Robert S. Meldelsohn, M.D., in *Confessions of a Medical Heretic* says that macrobiotics, on the other hand, incorporates diet in a "universal system of thought and behavior. It does not get caught in the trap of singling out cholesterol or vitamins or trace minerals or proteins. Macrobiotics is a synthesizing system. Modern nutrition in contrast depends on analysis . . . this often leads, as everyone knows, to paralysis by analysis."

However, as we aren't, many of us, familiar with Eastern philosophy and the "oneness of Tao," the final section is for those of us who are concerned about the possibility of not eating a properly balanced diet that contains all the necessary nutrients. There are many books on the subject, but this will, I hope, give a cross reference to which we analytical westerners can refer.

The Chemistry of Carbohydrates

The words *carbohydrates* and *starches* have an ominous ring to the ears of most figure-conscious bodies, although unrefined complex carbohydrates are reckoned to be the healthiest and best energy source we can have. Nan Bronfen, nutritionist for the Pritikin Research Foundation, says that grains and legumes should be our main calorie supply and adds, "Let me stress grains should be whole."

There are two principal kinds of carbohydrates: *complex carbohydrates* and *simple sugars*. To make them, plants need sunlight, carbon dioxide, and water.

Complex carbohydrates are constructed of many sugar units joined together. Before they can be used by the body, they must be broken down into one of the simplest sugars—*glucose*. This breaking down is done gradually by the enzymes in the mouth and digestive tract. This slow digestion means a steady, easily regulated flow of glucose into the bloodstream, for distribution as usable energy.

Simple sugars, however, are very different from complex carbohydrates in their effect on the body. They enter the bloodstream directly and quickly, causing a sudden rise in blood sugar and stimulating the pancreas to release insulin in large quantities. In time, as with an addictive drug, more and more may be needed to get that energy "high."

Some simple sugars are:

Sucrose: cane or beet, made up of glucose and fructose.

Fructose: found in fruits and vegetables.

Lactose: milk-sugar made up of galactose and glucose.

Maltose: freed by the digestion of starch. It consists of two glucose molecules.

Cellulose: a complex carbohydrate. Our body cannot use it for energy and it is often removed in food processing. However, although mainly indigestible, cellulose is vital to healthy digestion as a major part of roughage.

WHITE SUGAR

White sugar has been referred to as "pure, white, and deadly" and a "source of empty calories," providing energy and nothing else. The chemical reaction white sugar causes in the body gobbles up B vitamins and can lead to a calcium-phosphorus imbalance. Because of powerful publicity campaigns we feel it supplies "instant energy," but all foods contain calories. White sugar we can and should do without. It rots our teeth, makes us neurotic—and fat!

"If you look for sweetness," said Buddha, "your search will be endless, you will never be satisfied. But if you seek the true taste you will find what you are looking for."

MOLASSES

Molasses is the residue left after the extraction of sugar—or most of it—from the cane. Blackstrap molasses contains concentrates of iron, calcium, zinc, copper and chromium as well as lead, pesticides, and sulfur—ingredients not always mentioned on the label or in the food charts! It is in some ways the least wholesome of the products extracted from the sugarcane plant.

HONEY

Honey has less calories per weight than white sugar; otherwise it contains the same large amounts of fructose, glucose, and sucrose—and only slightly more vitamins and minerals.

Many claims are made that honey will cure arthritis, rheumatism, sleeplessness, and bedwetting, and that it will help sexual activities, restore sexual potency, and retard the aging process. There is, however, no scientific or nutritional basis for any such claims.

SACCHARINE AND SUGAR SUBSTITUTES

Such commercial products bear no relationship to natural sugar sweeteners, and there is continued concern about their long-term safety. (*See also* INGREDIENTS—Barley Malt, Carob, Rice Syrup, Maple Syrup.)

Facts About Fats

When we eat more food than we need—which is more often than not—our excess energy is stored as *fat*.

Fats are composed of the same three elements as carbohydrates: carbon, hydrogen, and oxygen. They are, though, a more concentrated form of energy. The fats and fatty substances in the body are called *lipids*. These are mainly composed from among some seventy or more different *fatty acids* plus *glycerol*. Fatty acids are either *saturated* or *unsaturated*. *Saturated* fats are solid at room temperature. *Unsaturated* fats tend to be liquid (oils) at room temperature.

Fats are absolutely necessary to us, but a diet high in fats encourages the body to make too much *cholesterol*.

CHOLESTEROL

Cholesterol is also a kind of *lipid*. The body produces plenty of its own cholesterol, and there is really no need to include it in the diet. Excess amounts can harden and block the arteries, which frequently leads to heart disease.

Cholesterol is found in most animal products but never in whole foods from plant sources. It is in all meats —particularly organ meats. Four ounces of liver, for example, contain three and a half times the maximum daily allowance! Eggs have 250 mg in each yolk, which is two and a half times this allowance. Full-fat dairy products are high in cholesterol. Whole milk is reputedly dangerous for anyone over two years of age!

LECITHIN

Lecithin is a lipid very similar in chemical composition to other fats. It is made in the body by the liver and consists of fatty acids and phosphates, which makes it both water and fat soluble.

Some nutritionists now say that it could cause the same problems as other fatty substances in the body. The use of lecithin as a supplement and additive is therefore not advised.

MARGARINE

To make margarine, unsaturated fats are saturated by adding hydrogen so that they will resemble the texture of butter. These altered, artificial fats lack vitamin E and linoleic acid (an essential fatty acid) and may also tend to increase the cholesterol and fats in the blood. Nickel is sometimes used as a catalyst and can remain in the product with possible harmful effects. Palm and coconut oils are often contained in cheaper margarines. These oils can be 99 percent saturated—which is more saturated than beef fat!

UNSATURATED OILS

Processed, refined oils have invariably been exposed to heat. Heat causes oxidation and destroys vitamin E. Such oils can oxidize easily in the body and thus destroy vitamins. When buying oils be sure they are as *unrefined* as possible and are cold pressed. Use them sparingly when cooking. Sauté at lower temperatures with less oil, or use water instead. (*See also* INGREDIENTS—Oils.)

Protein Complements

To make proteins, plants again use carbon, hydrogen, and oxygen with the addition of the important element nitrogen and sometimes sulfur. It is only by eating plants, or by eating animals that eat plants, that human and beast can obtain nitrogen.

And just as carbohydrates are built of sugar units and fats of fatty acids, proteins are made up of *amino acids*. *Amino* means "containing nitrogen in a certain form."

AMINO ACIDS—COMPLETE PROTEIN

Proteins are not used in the form in which we eat them. They are first broken down into twenty-two amino acids. The body is able to synthesize all of these except eight, which are therefore known as *essential* amino acids. Protein containing all eight of these is called *complete* protein.

COMPLEMENTARY PROTEINS

Some foods are high in certain essential amino acids and low in others. However, by combining a food low in one with food high in that particular amino acid, a more complete protein supply results. Grain and beans eaten together complement each other and can actually increase the percentage of usable protein by up to 40 percent, providing more protein than meat. The whole can thus be greater than the sum of its parts!

Complementary grain and bean diets have evolved and have been traditionally practiced by people all over the world. American Indians eat their corn or wheat tortillas and frijoles. Rice and beans are a popular staple in Jamaican and other Carribean island diets. Middle Easterners have chickpeas with their wheat couscous, and India is the country of chapati or rice and lentils. Indonesians cook tempeh, a soybean ferment, with their rice, and in China, Japan, and Korea other soy products—tofu, miso, and tamari—are served with rice. Macrobiotics uses all these various complements to boost protein supply.

Of all the nutrients in our diet, protein is probably the least likely to be deficient. Excessive amounts, on the other hand, can undoubtedly be harmful.

MEAT AS A SOURCE OF PROTEIN

There is generally a look of alarm and despondency on the faces of meat eaters when grains are suggested as an alternative principal food, but nutritionists give some pretty convincing reasons for not eating too much of this form of protein. Even athletes are often advised these days to use complex carbohydrates as a main source of energy.

Meat contains complete protein but not as much as is generally thought. Seventy to 80 percent of the calories in meat comes from fat, and meat is high in cholesterol.

These days many animals—cattle, pigs, chickens, turkeys—are treated with antibiotics to stimulate growth and resistance to disease in unsanitary, crowded conditions. It has been estimated that meat can contain the residues of up to 143 different drugs! The recent mad cow disease crisis also has led to a serious reassessment of what cattle are being fed.

Meat is, in fact, an elaborate and expensive way to obtain proteins. One nutritionist says, "It is time to drop the notion that we need meat to survive." Another says, "Grains and legumes will provide sufficient protein without all that extra fat."

Main Minerals

It is interesting that our body fluids, the very blood in our veins, resemble the mineral content of the ocean from which, we are told, life evolved. The enzymes and cells of our bodies depend on the major salts of the sea.

The body cannot manufacture its own minerals as it can some vitamins. They must be supplied by, and are available in, a proper diet. They should be taken in food rather than in extracted form as pills. Dr. William Strain of Cleveland has rather grimly likened element nutrition to a giant spider's web. If one strand of the web is pulled the whole structure is distorted!

Minerals are not destroyed by heat, light, or air. They can be lost from food in the cooking water—so always keep that water and use it! Minerals are usually extracted when foods are processed.

The Macronutrient Minerals

CALCIUM (CA)

We have two to three pounds of calcium in our body—it is the most abundant mineral—but only 20 to 30 percent of the amount ingested is used. Excessive consumption of meat, rich in phosphorus, upsets the calcium-phosphorus balance. A fatty diet interferes with calcium absorption.

Calcium and Exercise

Exercise—or the lack of it—is an important factor as exercise helps keep minerals in the bones, and weight-bearing movements cause calcium absorption into bone. Walking, running, and even light weight-training are recommended.

PHOSOPHORUS (P)

This, the second most abundant mineral in the body, makes up 1 percent of the human body weight—half that of calcium—90 percent of which is combined with oxygen as phosphates deposited in the bones and teeth. It depends on vitamin D and calcium for its absorption.

Excess intakes of iron, aluminum, and magnesium can interfere with phosphorus absorption, as they form insoluble phosphates. The calcium-phosphorus balance is disturbed by sugar intake or by high milk, fat, or protein diets.

Nan Bronfen says that modern humans are eating two or three times more phosphorus than calcium, which is the wrong balance. Plants and vegetables are fed with phosphate fertilizers and are sprayed with insecticides; phosphates are added to processed foods and sodas to give an acid flavor.

POTASSIUM (K)

Potassium is alkaline forming and is the third most plentiful mineral in the body. Most of it is used inside the body cells, while sodium is found in the fluids outside the cells. It works in constant dynamic balance with sodium throughout the body.

The average American's intake has been estimated at anything up to 6,000 mg, three times a suggested daily requirement, since the potassium content of many foods is high. Macrobiotics recommends moderate intakes with a sodium-potassium balance of 5:1 to 7:1. (*See also* YIN AND YANG.)

SODIUM (NA)

The unprocessed "salt of the earth" of ancient times and provider of a number of trace sea minerals has been commercially replaced, unfortunately, by "refined" table salt—pure sodium chloride. Most of the other natural salts of the sea have been extracted then iodine is added, sometimes sugar to make it pour, even sodium bicarbonate as a bleach to keep it white! Unrefined sea salt has a slightly off-white "glow" because of its mineral "impurity," which can be up to 12 percent. Sodium taken naturally with these minerals is not to be feared but respected.

Most people take far more sodium than they need, especially in refined salt. According to the *Manual of Nutrition*, published in London by HMSO, adults need 4 grams each day in a temperate climate, which can be achieved by eating natural food. Most people take in from 5 to 20 grams. Such excess sodium may cause potassium to be lost and is strongly associated with high blood pressure.

SULFUR (S)

Since early times people have visited mineral springs, or spas, to "take" waters that smell strongly of sulfur. Such water contains hydrogen sulfide. Suflur, like potassium, is found inside every body cell, especially in those of the hair. In fact, the smell of burning hair is due to a 15 percent sulfur content. Most of the peculiar odors of foods in the body laboratory are due to the presence of sulfur compounds! A diet containing enough protein will provide adequate sulfur.

CHLORINE (CL)

Chlorine is usually found in the body in some compound form with sodium or potassium as *chloride*. The total amount present is around 3 ounces. It is essential for the acid-alkaline balance in the blood and the production of hydrochloric acid in the stomach for digestion.

As sodium chloride in the form of table salt is widely distributed in our food there is no problem in obtaining sufficient amounts. The chlorine in drinking water can destroy vitamin E and impair the intestinal flora that helps digestion.

MAGNESIUM (MG)

Our body supply of magnesium is approximately 21 grams, 70 percent of which is located in the skeleton. It does not leave the bones as readily as do calcium and phosphorus.

Heavy drinkers, people living on refined foods, or those who drink soft water, are apt to have a low magnesium supply. The milling process removes 86 percent of it from white flour, and refined grains increase the body's need for magnesium, which is essential to carbohydrate metabolism.

The U.S. Research Council's recommended daily intake is 350 mg for men, 300 for women, and 450 during pregnancy, which the average refined food diet will barely provide.

The Trace Elements

IRON (FE)

In your body there are a mere 3 to 4 grams of the same mineral used to make your cast-iron skillet, but without this iron life would cease in a few seconds! Iron lies at the center of a large and complex protein molecule, *hemoglobin*, which transports oxygen to the cells of the body. Without oxygen no energy is released.

Poor eating habits and preserved foods that have been depleted of iron can lessen supplies, as can eating too many sweets. Eggs seem to decrease the amount of iron absorbed, taking alkaline indigestion cures, drinking too much coffee and tea all hinder absorption. Sea vegetables are an exceptionally rich source of iron.

There is so much more attention given to iron deficiency, which is only one form of anemia, than iron overload, often caused by years of iron tonics or large volumes of iron-containing wines. It tends to occur mostly in men over forty. Symptoms include loss of weight and a gray pallor to the skin.

IODINE (I)

The content of trace elements in foods often depends on the soil in which plants are grown. In the early 1900s, for instance, the soil of the Midwest and Great Lakes areas in the United States was deficient in iodine and this became known as the Goiter Belt. People living in certain areas around the world often had a high incidence of enlarged thyroid glands. Today food sold in markets is usually from many different areas. Sea vegetables, however, are always a rich and reliable source of iodine.

Iodine, as a constituent of *thyroxine*, assists in regulating the body's energy. Cretinism can be the result of a limited iodine intake by the mother during pregnancy.

MANGANESE (MN)

Manganese is described as one of the "desirable" elements. It plays a role in activating numerous enzymes in the body. The main food sources of manganese are from whole grains, nuts, and vegetables. Manganese is often removed from the soil by lime that is added to increase vegetable foliage. Milling of grain also removes manganese; corn, for instance, contains 1 mg per 100 g and corn flakes only 0.04 mg.

COPPER (CU)

There is evidence that copper should be classified as a "heavy metal," as are lead, mercury, and cadmium. It is essential to the body, however, in very small amounts. As iron metabolism is highly dependent on it, copper is important for the proper formation of hemoglobin.

Copper is present in many foods, especially whole grains, beans, nuts, and seafood. Deficiency is usually due to excessive intake of certain other minerals (for example, by supplementation). The proportion of copper to these other minerals, particularly zinc, is important. High doses of vitamin C can interfere with its absorption.

Toxicity from excess copper is rare but copper cooking utensils should always be lined with stainless steel.

ZINC (ZN)

Zinc, which is related to the normal absorption and action of vitamins, especially the B complex, maintains about twenty enzyme systems in the body and is described as the "traffic policeman," directing and overseeing the efficient flow of these body processes. It is readily absorbed in the body and is found in the male reproductive fluid. The prostate gland contains more zinc than any other part of the body, and delayed sexual maturity in adolescents has recently been connected with zinc deficiency. Stretch marks on the skin and white spots in the finger nails may indicate zinc deficiency.

Apart from soil exhaustion, the most common cause of poor zinc supply is that food processing removes zinc—bugs cannot grow without zinc either!—while soluble zinc salts can go down the drain with the vegetable water. Pregnant women and those on the "pill" can have low zinc levels while foods high in copper can negate much of the zinc obtained. Oysters, for instance, are very high in zinc but are also high in copper!

How Vital Are Vitamins?

Nature makes most vitamins from carbon, hydrogen, and oxygen in differing proportions. Around twenty vitamins have so far been identified, but not all are scientifically or officially accepted or understood.

In 1912 a substance was discovered in the polishings from whole grain or "brown" rice that prevented beriberi. It was called *thiamine—amine* means "containing nitrogen." The word *vitamine*, as it was originally spelled, meant *vita* (life) and *amine* (nitrogenous). By the 1920s, however, the *e* was dropped as very few vitamins proved to contain nitrogen.

Although the thiamine in whole grain rice has been known to prevent beriberi for many years, polished white rice, minus its supply of thiamine, continues to be the staple human food of the Far East, and beriberi continues to be a widespread deficiency disease there. In the Western world, white refined bread and white refined flour are our main cereal food. Vitamins and minerals are often completely removed from them and we are encouraged to make up the deficiencies in our diets by taking supplement tablets invariably manufactured, at huge profit, from the very nutrients that have been taken from our grains in the first place!

Vitamins are essential factors needed for the healthy functioning of the body, but supplementation with isolated vitamins is regarded with suspicion. Nan Bronfen says categorically that vitamins, when used in their extracted forms rather than as parts of whole foods, are being used as drugs. An overdose of one vitamin can increase the deficiency of others because of their complex interrelationships. Vitamins are interdependent, and nature knows best how to package them.

Some vitamins are soluble in water—the B complex vitamins and vitamin C—others are fat soluble—these are vitamins A, D, E, F, and K. Some are resistant to heat, some are not; some are destroyed by storage, light, air, acid, alkali, pollution, processing, and cooking in copper or aluminum. Alcohol, smoking, stress, and "the pill" can all increase the body's need for vitamins. It is important to be aware of the losses that occur when cooking: prolonged boiling of vegetables in water leaches out water-soluble vitamins. Place vegetables in boiling water—not too much of it—to "seal" them. Keep the cooking water, and use it for soup stock or to make sauces—or drink it! It's usually delicious, particularly if seasoned with a little tamari or miso. Avoid cooking vegetables too long.

VITAMIN A

The functions of vitamin A in the body are, it is generally admitted, not completely understood. Plant foods do not contain vitamin A, but a substance called *ß-carotene* (as in carrots), which is readily converted into vitamin A by the body. Orange-colored or dark green vegetables and orange-colored fruit contain especially plentiful supplies of ß-carotene. Carotene is stored in the body fat and overdosing can turn the skin yellow.

Vitamin A is good for eye conditions and proper night vision. Working in bright light, dim light, or fluorescent light raises the body's demand for it as does TV, some drugs, smoking, car fumes, and air pollution. Older people, who especially need green vegetables, often consume too few.

THE B-COMPLEX VITAMINS

Scientific understanding of the relationship between diet and nervous and psychotic disorders is in its infancy, but it is realized that the B vitamins are related to mental health, nerve cell and tissue functioning, as well as the metabolism of carbohydrates, amino acids, and fats. B vitamins are difficult to separate and, though seemingly independent, each has a specific, related function. They are supplied mainly by the same whole foods: whole grains, legumes, land vegetables, sea vegetables, nuts, and seeds. Meats and liver, which are extreme yang, also contain B vitamins. Brewers yeast and molasses are also considered good sources, but they are extreme yin.

B vitamins are, as we have said, frequently removed from whole foods by refining processes to "improve" color and texture and to "curtail pest attraction." The pests, quite rightly, don't like refined foods! Sugar, alcohol, and oral contraceptives also increase the need for B vitamins.

VITAMIN B$_1$ (THIAMINE)

Thiamine, the magic ingredient discovered in rice polishings, was the first member of the B complex to be chemically identified. It contains sulfur as well as nitrogen and is highly soluble in water, which means it has limited body storage and needs to be supplied daily.

Thiamine is part of an enzyme complex needed to metabolize carbohydrates into simple sugar for energy production. It is essential for the health of the nervous system and is consequently known as the morale vitamin because of its beneficial effect on mental attitudes. It can help prevent travel sickness.

Heat and hot water cause loss of vitamin B$_1$. Never overcook vegetables or throw out the cooking water. Body supplies are depleted by excessive sugar intake, smoking, and drinking alcohol. Thiamine can also be destroyed by an enzyme present in raw clams and oysters. It is inhibited by caffeine, food processing methods, and "the pill."

VITAMIN B$_2$ (RIBOFLAVIN)

Vitamin B$_2$ is reported to be one of the most commonly deficient vitamins in America. Most common symptoms are: cracks and lesions in the corner of the mouth; inflamed, sore tongue; itching and burning of the eyes; eye fatigue; sensitivity to light; dermatitis around the nose, mouth, forehead, and ears. Deficiency symptoms of various B vitamins are often so similar however that it is sometimes difficult to tell which is lacking. Large supplementary doses of any of them may result in high losses. Light, especially ultraviolet light, destroys it and alkaline solutions (baking soda), sulfur drugs, alcohol, and "the pill" increase demands.

VITAMIN B_3 (NIACIN)

During famines caused by the Napoleonic wars, farmers in Europe, living almost entirely on corn, were stricken by an epidemic of a dreadful skin and nerve disease called pellagra. Even today corn is used mainly as animal food in Europe because of its grim association with the disease. The missing nutrient from corn proved to be *niacin*. Corn does contain all the B vitamins, but the niacin is not released in the body. Indians in Mexico and Peru have eaten beans with their corn since ancient times and have supplemented their diet in this way. Niacin is fairly stable but excessive consumption of sugar and alcohol, certain antibiotics, and sleeping tablets deplete the body's supply—as does "the pill."

VITAMIN B_5 (PANTOTHENIC ACID)

The Greek word *panthos* means "everywhere." *Pantothenic acid*, or vitamin B_5, occurs in all living cells and was first isolated in Texas in 1940. It affects all manner of bodily chemical functions, is water soluble, and synthesized by bacterial flora of the intestines.

Pantothenic acid is so widely distributed that an isolated deficiency of vitamin B_5 from among other B complex vitamins is rare, and the means of detecting it are limited.

VITAMIN B_6 (PYRIDOXINE)

In the 1930s a factor was discovered in animal liver that prevented skin disorders in rats and also in humans. Vitamin B_6 consists of three related compounds: *pyridoxine, pyridoxinal,* and *pyridoxamine*. It is water soluble but stable to heat, light, air and acid and is needed for the proper absorption of vitamin B_{12}. Another of its functions is to help maintain the balance of sodium and potassium that regulates the body fluids.

The need for it increases during pregnancy, lactation, aging, and if taking oral contraceptives. The consumption of protein also increases the demand for vitamin B_6. Deficiency symptoms are similar to those of vitamins B_2 and B_3: numbness and cramps in arms and legs, tingling hands, cracks around the mouth and eyes, nervousness, and depression.

VITAMIN B_{12} (COBALAMIN)

Vitamin B_{12} is the first cobalt-containing substance found necessary for life and the only vitamin containing an essential mineral element. It cannot be made synthetically, but can be produced by fermentation.

Vegetarian diets are frequently high in folic acid, which may mask a vitamin B_{12} deficiency; serious nerve damage and pernicious anemia could result. Vegans, who eat no meat, fish, or dairy products, need to be sure they have some sea vegetables, miso, or tempeh as these are good sources of the vitamin (*see* INGREDIENTS—Miso and Tempeh). Absorption increases during pregnancy and decreases with age. Impaired memory and concentration in older people may often be caused by a lack of vitamin B_{12}. Amounts required are minute but essential.

FOLIC ACID: FOLACIN

Folic acid, also known as vitamin M or Bm was first isolated from the leaf vegetable spinach. It works closely with vitamin B_{12} and excessive supplementation of it can disguise the symptoms of vitamin B_{12} deficiency and of pernicious anemia.

Folic acid is lost in food refining and processing. A major cause of folic acid deficiency is destruction during prolonged cooking, refrigeration, or storage at room temperature in the light for long periods. Excess alcohol, chlorine in drinking water, antibiotics, and "the pill" all increase requirements. Deficiency is common among the elderly and people who eat too few green leafy vegetables. Adequate folic acid consumption is important during pregnancy.

VITAMIN C (ASCORBIC ACID)

As early as 1747 a British physician, James Lind, M.D. (1716–1794), discovered that lime juice prevented the scurvy that had plagued sailors of that time. Boiling the lime juice with water destroyed the effect of the nourishing factor. This factor was vitamin C, a sugarlike substance that most animals can synthesize in their bodies from glucose, the exceptions being monkeys, guinea pigs, the Indian fruit bat, the red-vented bulbul bird apparently, and humans! Scurvy is still found today in older people living on convenience and junk foods.

Ascorbic acid, available in synthetic form, is the subject of argument as a possible cure for the common cold. Massive doses of it are recommended by some nutritionists and suspected by others. "Vitamin C can perhaps reduce the severity of a cold, but it may make it last longer!" says Nan Bronfen. It is much better to get it from whole foods than from pills, because foods containing the vitamin provide bioflavonoids, which protect it from oxidation. Vitamin C is the least stable vitamin; it is very sensitive to oxygen and its potency is lost through exposure to light, heat, and air. It is very water soluble and, although readily absorbed, most of it is eliminated in three or four hours.

The body's ability to absorb vitamin C is reduced by smoking (one cigarette can use up to 25 mg), air pollution, and alcohol. As vitamin C is needed for adrenalin production it is used up more rapidly under stress or shock. The ingestion of aspirin, pain killers, sulfur drugs, antibiotics, and cortisone increases demands. Baking soda creates an alkaline medium, which destroys it, and cooking in copper or aluminum is also destructive. Drinking too much water will deplete the body's vitamin C.

The recommended daily amount required is around 45 mg for adults, preferably taken in frequent small doses.

VITAMIN D

This, the "sunshine vitamin," is really a hormone needed only in miniscule amounts and is made by the body. Ultraviolet light from the sun converts a type of cholesterol called ergosterol in the skin into vitamin D, which is absorbed into the circulatory system. The body can store sizable reserves of it. Very small areas of skin need to be exposed, as 18 International Units per square centimeter can be manufactured in three hours! Pigmentation is a factor—the more pigment there is, the less vitamin D is produced. Deficiency can cause faulty mineralization of bones, which can lead to rickets. There is a risk that children of dark-skinned immigrants to a northern climate may develop rickets from lack of sunlight as their skin prevents them from producing vitamin D as readily as do light-skinned people. Vitamin D is not lost in the cooking water but is lost in the oil when frying! Provitamins D are found also in both plant and animal tissue. Foods containing vitamin A usually contain some vitamin D.

VITAMIN E (TOCOPHEROL)

This fat-soluble vitamin is composed of a group of seven substances called *tocopherols*. Of these *alphatocopherol* is the most potent and valuable form of vitamin E found in oil-containing foods such as grains, seeds, and nuts as well as leafy greens and fish.

Fats and oils containing vitamin E are less susceptible to oxidation or rancidity than are those without it. The cosmetic industry claims that vitamin E can help retard the ageing process and it is often used, in ointment form, on the skin.

Vitamin E is destroyed by processing. White flour, for instance, no longer contains much vitamin E as the germ of the wheat, which is the richest known source, is removed. W. E. Shute, M.D , a leading heart specialist, claims that "prior to the removal of natural wheat germ, with its vitamin E, from whole wheat flour and bread there were no cases of coronary thrombosis; now it is one of the world's major killers." A diet high in refined vegetable oils and polyunsaturated fats and oils increases the demand for vitamin E. Chlorine in drinking water, rancid oil or fat, inorganic iron supplements, air pollution, and mineral oil used as a laxative, all deplete supplies. "The pill" neutralizes the effect of vitamin E, and air pollution increases the need for it.

Women severely deficient in vitamin E are likely to have fertility problems, and men can be made sterile.

Chief Food Sources Table

An indication of some of the chief food sources of vitamins and minerals. Quantities shown are per 100 grams.

VITAMIN A (i.u.): Red pepper 21,600; dandelion green 14,000; carrot 11,000; kale 10,000; parsley 8,500; spinach 8,000; Swiss chard 6,500; chives 5,800; watercress 4,900; broccoli 2,500; onion 40; pumpkin 1,600; nori 11,000; kombu 430; apricot 2,700 (dried 10,000); cantaloupe 3,400; cod liver oil 85,000; crab 2,170.

VITAMIN B_1 (mg): Millet 0.73; brown rice 0.35; wheat 0.57; rye 0.43; soybean 1.10; aduki 0.50; lentils 0.37; peanuts 1.14; Brazil nut 0.96; chestnut 0.32; sunflower seed 1.96; sesame seed 0.98; pumpkin seed 0.24; nori 0.25; burdock 0.30; gingerroot 0.20; brewer's yeast 4.46.

VITAMIN B_2 (mg): Millet 0.38; rye 0.22; corn 0.12; wheat 0.12; brown rice 0.05; lentils 0.22; soybean 0.13; aduki 0.1; nori 1.24; kelp 0.33; kombu 0.32; mushroom 0.46; turnip greens 0.39; burdock 0.3; kale 0.26; parsley 0.26; broccoli 0.23; almond 0.92; sunflower seed 0.23; brewer's yeast 4.28.

VITAMIN B_3 (mg): Brown rice 4.7; durum wheat/buckwheat 4.4; wheat 4.3; barley 3.7; millet 2.3; dried peas 3.0; aduki 2.5; soybean 2.2 (tempeh 2.52); peanuts 17.2; sesame seed 5.4; sunflower seed 5.4; almond 2.5; green pea 2.9; kale 2.1; parsley 1.2; nori 10; wakame 10; kelp 5.7; mackerel 8.4; salmon 7.2; sardine 5.4; trout 8.4; brewer's yeast 37.9.

VITAMIN B_5 (mg): Mushroom 2.2; cabbage 1.63; cauliflower 1.00; kale 1.00; parsnip 0.6; squash 0.36; parsley 0.3; brown rice 1.07; bulgur wheat 0.65; corn (cooked) 0.44; peas 0.75; pinto bean 0.65; blackeyed peas 0.4; almond 4.7; sunflower seed 1.37; cashew 1.3; walnut 0.9; chestnut 0.5; avocado 1.07; dates 0.78; blackcurrant 0.4; trout 1.96; swordfish 1.95; lobster 1.5; salmon 1.3; brewer's yeast 12.5.

VITAMIN B_6 (mg): Buckwheat 0.57; brown rice 0.55; pearled barley 0.22; soybean 0.81 (tempeh 0.85); pinto bean 0.5; lima 0.17; nori 1.04; kombu 0.87; kale 0.3; spinach 0.26; brussels sprouts 0.23; carrot 0.15; sunflower seed 1.25; walnut 0.73; chestnut 0.33; banana 0.51; avocado 0.42; raisins 0.24; salmon 0.70; rainbow trout 0.69; mackerel 0.66; brewer's yeast 2.5.

VITAMIN B_{12} (mcg): Oysters 18.0; crab 10.0; herring 9.0; mackerel 9.0; trout 5.7; salmon 3.5; haddock 1.3; nori 21; ulva 6.3; hijiki 0.57; kombu 0.3; tempeh 3.9; beef liver 79.9; eggs 1.54; low fat milk 0.46; yogurt 0.42; brie 1.37; gruyere 1.36.

FOLIC ACID (mcg): Bulgur wheat 4.70; brown rice 20; wheat 10; chickpea 200; pinto bean 200; soybean 100; blackeyed peas 100; fenugreek 5,700; peanuts 150; almond 130; pumpkin seed 140; hazelnut 90; spinach 190; parsley 140; brussels sprouts 80; broccoli 70; cauliflower 55 (cooked 35); watercress 50; hijiki 20; nori 10; orange 40; avocado 50; pear 14; dates 20; liver 300.

VITAMIN C (mg): Red pepper 369; kale 186; parsley 172; turnip tops 136; broccoli 113; brussels sprouts 102; watercress 79; cauliflower 78; lotus root 75; chives 56; spinach 51; cabbage 47; onion 31; bean sprouts 20; acerola cherry 1,300; guava 242; blackcurrant 200; orange 77; strawberry 49.

VITAMIN D (mcg): Food containing Vitamin A; kippers 1,000; mackerel 700; sardines 300; tuna 232; cod 100 (cod liver oil 8,400); shiitake mushrooms 2,639.

VITAMIN E (mg): Millet 1.75; brown rice 1.53; cucumber 8.4; kale 8.0; turnip greens 2.3; spinach 2.27; peas 2.1; Swiss chard 1.5; lettuce 0.4; hazelnut 20.7; pecan 15.0; brazil 6.5; mango 1.0; apple 0.7; bananas 0.4; strawberry 0.4; wheat germ oil 153.6; corn oil 78.5; safflower oil 75.0; soybean oil 56.4; sesame oil 16.4; sunflower oil 9.3; herring 2.0; mackerel 1.6; cod liver oil 25.7.

CALCIUM (mg): Hijiki 1,400; wakame 1,300; arame 1,170; kelp 1,093; parsley 203; carrot top 203; watercress 150; broccoli 103; buckwheat 114; oats 55; brown rice 52; soybean 226; chickpea 150; sesame seed 1,160; hazelnut 209; sardines 437; milk 118.

PHOSPHORUS (mg): Pumpkin seed 1,144; sunflower seed 837; sesame seed 616; arame 616; nori 510; dulse 267; wheat 410; brown rice 377; rye 376; oats 320; aduki 350; lentils 377; sardine 459; snapper 214; cod 194; chicken 220; beef 155.

POTASSIUM (mg): Dulse 8,071; kombu 6,600; kelp 5,273; nori 3,800; soybean 1,677; aduki 1,500; pinto bean 984; chickpea 797; sunflower seed 920; almond 778; sesame seed 725; parsley 727; parsnip 540; Swiss chard 550; garlic 529; spinach 470; dried banana 1,477; prunes 700; raisins 763; rye 467; millet 430; wheat 370; cod 382; snapper 323.

SODIUM (mg): Kelp 3,007; Irish moss 2,892; kombu 2,500; olive 800; beet greens 130; celery 126; daikon 100; spinach 71; kale 75; lentils 30; chickpea 26; aduki 20; sesame seed 60; sunflower seed 30; oats 10; brown rice 9; sardine 823; oyster 121; cod 70; beef 67.

SULFUR (mg): Kale 8,600; watercress 5,351; brussels sprouts 3,530; cabbage 1,710; turnip 1,210; carrot 445; onion 265; kelp 930; peach 350; raisins 255; watermelon 210; strawberry 205; apple 201; soybean 263; lima 260; lentils 120; sweet corn 240; barley 240; rye 28; brown rice 10; shrimp 339; haddock 238; red salmon 226; trout 224; eggs 197.

CHOLINE (mg): Celery 1,780; lettuce 1,382; spinach 1,130; red cabbage 1,051; kale 1,050; cabbage 1,045; parsnip 1,040; kelp 1,221; lentils 150; chickpea 95; soybean 40; sunflower seed 90; Brazil nut 85; walnut 12; dates 390; raspberry 290; blackberry 180; barley 35; wheat 7; rice 2.

MAGNESIUM (mg): Kelp 760; dulse 220; soybeans 265; lima 180; dried peas 180; lentils 80; millet 162; wheat 160; rye 115; brown rice 88; almond 270; sesame seed 181; spinach 88; Swiss chard 65; parsley 41; kale 37; carrot 23; onion 12; dried banana 132; avocado 45; blackberry 30.

IRON (mg): Dulse 150; nori 106; kelp 100; hijiki 29; kombu 15; millet 6.8; oats 4.5; rye 3.7; buckwheat 3.1; chickpea 6.9; lentils 6.8; soybeans 6.4; parsley 6.2; red pepper 6.2; beet greens 3.3; chard 3.2; spinach 3.1; pumpkin seed 11.2; sesame seed 10.5; thyme 123; cumin seed 66.2; dried apricot 5.5; brewer's yeast 17.5.

IODINE (mg): Kombu 193; kelp 150; arame 98; shellfish 0.29; Swiss chard 0.099; turnip greens 0.076; squash 0.062; onion 0.014; carrot 0.012: watermelon 0.04; strawberry 0.019; peach 0.016; apple 0.009; peanut 0.02; walnut 0.003; brown rice 0.002.

MANGANESE (mg): Wheat 5; oats 3; brown rice 2; barley 1.7; buckwheat 1.3; turnip greens 1.4; beet 0.94; leeks 0.7; onions 0.6; parsley 0.6; kale 0.5; greens 0.4; carrot 0.1; ginger 17; avocado 2.0; blackcurrant 0.78; blackberry 0.63; hazelnut 4.2; chestnut 3.7; snail 1.6; oyster 0.2; egg 0.05.

COPPER (mg): Barley 0.4; brown rice 0.28; soybean 1.17; kidney bean 0.85; lima 0.73; mushroom 1.54; spinach 0.58; beet 0.22; squash 0.17; onion 0.15; carrot 0.15; sunflower seed 1.77; sesame seed 1.59; walnut 1.39; almond 1.03; avocado 0.4; raisins 0.25; lobster 2.2; crab 1.3.

ZINC (mg): Corn 2.5; brown rice 1.84; chickpea 2.7; blackeyed peas 1.0; lentils 1.0 (sprouted 1.5); Brazil nut 5.1; cashew 4.4; hazelnut 3.0; caraway seed 5.7; basil 3.3; mushroom 1.3; spinach 0.91; cabbage 0.43; sauerkraut 0.8; carrot 0.4; peach 1.74; avocado 0.35; wheat germ 14.3; milk 3.8.

Appendix

Yin and Yang

UNIVERSAL PRINCIPLES*

- That which has a beginning has an end.

- Each thing is individual and unique.

- There can be no front without a back, no beauty without ugliness. Your opponent is your greatest benefactor. Sickness is the other side of health, for the back is the real meaning of the front.

- The greater and wider the front, the greater and wider the back. The greater the beauty, the greater the ugliness.

- All opposites are complementary and can be classified in two categories—yin and yang.

Acid- and Alkaline-Forming Foods

In an attempt to reconcile the Western concept of acid- and alkaline-forming foods with the Eastern Tao concept of yin-yang, Herman Aihara produced a chart (see overleaf) of four categories balancing yin and yang acid- and alkaline-forming foods.

Yang alkaline-forming foods are high in *sodium.*

Yang acid-forming foods are high in *phosphorus, sulfur,* and *sodium.*

Yin alkaline-forming foods are high in *potassium, magnesium,* and *calcium.*

Yin acid-forming foods are high in *phosphorus* and *sulfur.*

A meal should contain a selection of one food from each category. Grains, of course, should be the principal food (yang, acid forming) with vegetables—including sea vegetables—(yin, alkaline forming) and beans (yin, acid forming) with sesame salt, tamari, and salted pickles (yin, alkaline forming). This menu should be a balance of the acid-alkaline factors. It is always advisable to avoid eating extremes of acid and alkaline or yin and yang too often.

---

*Adapted from G. Ohsawa's *Zen Macrobiotics* and Michio Kushi's *Book of Macrobiotics.*

Barley

Yin Acid-Forming Foods

High in phosphorus and sulfur

sugar
sweets, candy
soft drinks
vinegar
saccharine
vodka
some wine
whiskey
sake
beer
soybeans
green peas
tofu
white beans
pinto beans
kidney beans
black beans
chickpeas
red beans (aduki)
macaroni
spaghetti

cashews
peanuts
almonds
chesnuts

corn oil
olive oil
sesame oil
peanut butter
sesame cream

Yang Acid-Forming Foods

High in phosphorus, sulfur, and sodium

corn, oats
barley, rye
wheat
rice
buckwheat

shellfish
eel, carp
white fish
cheese
fowl
meat
tuna, salmon
eggs

Yin Alkaline-Forming Foods

High in potassium, magnesium, and calcium

natural wine
natural sake
cola
cocoa
fruit juices
coffee
dyed teas
mineral waters
soda water
well water

honey
mustard
ginger
pepper
curry
cinnamon

tropical fruit
dates, figs
lemons, grapes
raisins, bananas
peaches
currants
pears, plums
oranges
watermelon

apples, cherries
strawberries

potatoes
eggplant
tomatoes
shiitake
taro potatoes
cucumber
sweet potatoes
mushrooms
spinach
asparagus
broccoli
celery
cabbage
pumpkin
onions
turnips
daikon
nori
hijiki
carrots

Yang Alkaline-Forming Foods

High in sodium

kuzu tea

millet

dandelion tea
mu tea
Ohsawa coffee
yannoh
ginseng

sesame salt
soy sauce
miso
umeboshi
salt

wakame
kombu
lotus root
burdock
dandelion root
jinenjo

Bibliography

Abehsera, Michel. *Zen Macrobiotic Cooking*. New York: Albyn Press, 1971.

———. *Cooking for Life*. Binghamton, N.Y.: Swan House, 1970.

Agriculture, U.S. Dept. of. *Handbook of Nutritional Contents of Foods*. New York: Dover Publications, 1975.

Aihara, Herman. *Acid & Alkaline*. Oroville, Calif.: Ohsawa Foundation, 1980.

———. *Seven Macrobiotic Principles*. Oroville, Calif.: Ohsawa Foundation, 1977.

Airola, Dr. Paavo. *Are You Confused?* Phoenix, Arizona: Health Plus Publishers, 1971.

Arasaki, S., and T. Arasaki. *Vegetables from the Sea*. Tokyo: Japan Publications, 1983.

Bethel, Mary. *The Healing Power of Herbs*. Wilshire Book Co., 1980.

Bronfen, Nan. *Nutrition for a Better Life*. Santa Barbara: Capra Press, 1980.

Caine, Mary. *The Glastonbury Giants*. Kingston, Surrey: Helios Books.

Clark, Linda. *Know Your Nutrition*. New Canaan: Keats. 1973.

Cooper, J. C. *Yin & Yang*. Wellingborough: Aquarian Press, 1981.

Detrick, Mia. *Sushi*. New York: Chronicle Books.

Dieno, Konrad, ed. *Documenta Geigy Scientific Tables*. Sydney, Australia: Geigy Pharmaceutical Pty. Ltd., 1983.

Douell and Bailey. *Cook's Ingredients*. New York: W. Morrow & Co. Inc., 1980.

Esko, Wendy. *Introducing Macrobiotic Cooking*. Tokyo: Japan Publications, 1983.

Esko, Edward, and Wendy Esko. *Macrobiotic Cooking for Everyone*. Tokyo: Japan Publications, 1980.

Ford Heritage BSME. *Composition & Facts About Foods*. Mokelumne Hill, Calif.: Health Research, 1971.

Holford, Patrick. *The Whole Health Manual*. Wellingborough: Thorsons, 1983.

Horn, Ken. *Chinese Cookery*. London: BBC, 1984.

Kinsman, Lisa. *Chinese Delights*. Norman & Hobhouse.

Kirschmann, John D. *Nutrition Almanac*. (Rev. ed.). New York: McGraw Book Company, 1979.

Kushi, Michio. *Cancer Prevention Diet*. New York: St. Martins Press, 1983.

———. *Macrobiotics Experience*. Brookline, Mass.: East West Foundation, 1975.

———. *The Order of the Universe Magazine*. Boston: Order of the Universe Publications, 1967.

Oats

Law, Donald. *You Are How You Eat*. Wellingborough, England: Turnstone, 1977.

Levine Gelb, Barbara. *Food & What's in It for You*. New York: Ballantine Books, 1980.

Mackarness, Dr Richard. *Not All in the Mind*. London: Pan, 1976.

Magnin, Pierre. *Macrobiotic Health Food*. Lima Publications, 1980.

Mervyn, Leonard. *Dictionary of Vitamins*. London: Thorsons, 1984.

Mindell, Earl. *Vitamin Bible*. New York: Warner Books, 1979.

Moore Lappe, Frances. *Diet for a Small Planet*. New York: Ballantine Books, 1975.

Ohsawa, George. *Zen Macrobiotics*. Los Angeles, New York: Ohsawa Foundation, 1965.

———. *Book of Judgement*. Los Angeles, New York: Ohsawa Foundation, 1966.

———. *Guide Book for Living*. Los Angeles, New York: Ohsawa Foundation, 1967.

———. *Macrobiotics: An Invitation to Health & Happiness*. San Francisco: Ohsawa Foundation, 1971.

Oles, Shayne. *The New Zen Cookery*. Woodland Hills, Calif.: Shayfer Corporation.

Peterson, Vicki. *The Natural Food Catalogue*. London & Sydney: Macdonald & Co., 1984.

Pfeiffer, Carl C. *Mental & Elemental Nutrients*. New Canaan: Keats Publishing Inc., 1975.

Polunin, Oleg, and Anthony Huxley. *Flowers of the Mediterranean*. London: Chatto & Windus, 1981.

Rawson, Philip, and Laszlo Legez. *Tao*. London: Thames & Hudson, 1973.

Rombauer, Irma, Marion Rombauer Becker, and Ethan Becker. *The Joy of Cooking*. New York: Scribner, 1997.

Sams, Craig. *About Macrobiotics*. London: Thorsons, 1983.

Scott, David. *Middle Eastern Vegetarian Cookery*. Melbourne, Aust.: Rider, 1982.

Sekules, Veronica. *Friends of the Earth Cookbook*. Harmondsworth, Middx.: Penguin, 1981.

Shurtleff, William, and Akiko Aoyagi. *The Book of Tofu*. Autumn Press, 1975.

———. *The Book of Miso*. Kanagawa-Ken, Japan: Autumn Press, 1976.

———. *The Book of Tempeh*. New York: Harper & Row, 1979.

Smith, Loudon. *Feed Yourself Right*. New York: McGraw-Hill, 1980.

Teitel, Martin, and Kimberly A. Wilson. *Genetically Engineered Food: Changing the Nature of Nature*. Rochester, Vt.: Park Street Press, 1999.

Thorpe, Susan. *The Four Seasons Wholefood Cookbook*. London: Thorsons, 1983.

Weber, Marcea. *Whole Meals*. Chalmington, Dorset: Prism Press, 1983.

Wheatley, Michael. *A Way of Living as a Means of Survival*. London: Corgi Books, 1977.

Index

Index

Index

Index